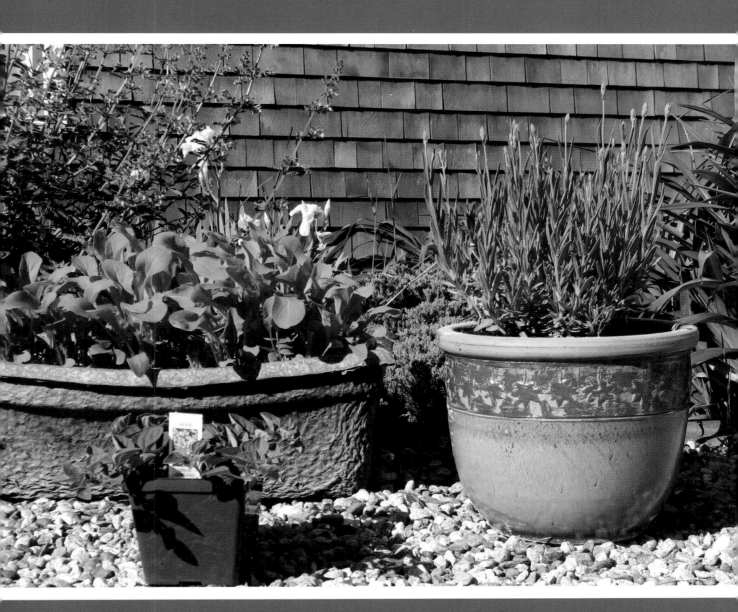

Published by Advantage, Charleston, South Carolina.
Member of Advantage Media Group.

ADVANTAGE is a registered trademark and the Advantage colophon is a trademark of Advantage Media Group, Inc.

Printed in the United States of America.

ISBN: 978-1-59932-644-3
LCCN: 2015958934
Photos courtesy of Donna Lind Photography: Cover photo, back flap, and pages 6, 12, 32, 36, 43, 44, 65, 73, 97, 98, 101, 115, 148, and 156.
Photos courtesy of Gina Lugo: pages 89, 142, and 145.
All other photos by Suzanne Sweeney.

This publication is designed to provide accurate and authoritative information in regard to the subject matter covered. It is sold with the understanding that the publisher is not engaged in rendering legal, accounting, or other professional services. If legal advice or other expert assistance is required, the services of a competent professional person should be sought.

Advantage Media Group is proud to be a part of the Tree Neutral® program. Tree Neutral offsets the number of trees consumed in the production and printing of this book by taking proactive steps such as planting trees in direct proportion to the number of trees used to print books. To learn more about Tree Neutral, please visit **www.treeneutral.com**. To learn more about Advantage's commitment to being a responsible steward of the environment, please visit **www.advantagefamily.com/green**

Advantage Media Group is a publisher of business, self-improvement, and professional development books and online learning. We help entrepreneurs, business leaders, and professionals share their Stories, Passion, and Knowledge to help others Learn & Grow. Do you have a manuscript or book idea that you would like us to consider for publishing? Please visit **advantagefamily.com** or call **1.866.775.1696**.

The information in this book is for informative purposes only and is the informed opinion of the author. This book is designed to help you make better-informed decisions about the food you eat. It is not intended nor should it be treated as a definitive guide on health and wellness, nor should it be regarded as medical or nutritional advice. The author is not liable for your use of the ideas presented in this book; neither will she be held responsible for any health problem, loss, damage, claim, or action that may result from the use of the information contained in this book. Readers are advised to consult their own health practitioners, doctors, or physicians for professional advice on matters relating to their health and well-being.

the

Optimal Health
Cookbook

Your Guide to Real Food
Made Easy

SUZANNE SWEENEY

Advantage

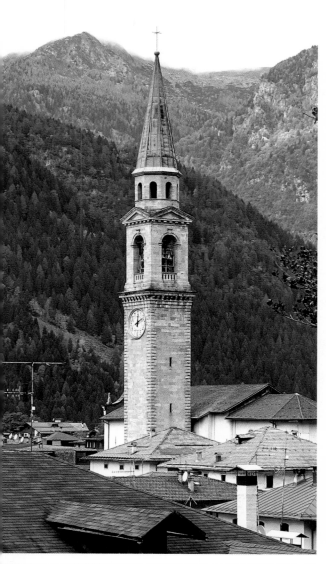

This book is dedicated to my

dear friend Mary.

We shared stories,

adventures, bragging rights to

our Italian heritage,

and many laughs.

Mary always had enough

for everyone.

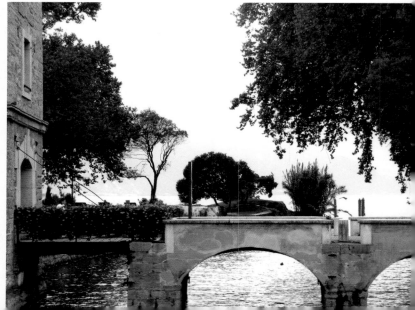

"Being a working mom with a toddler at home makes cooking healthy, delicious meals seem exhausting. Suzanne's recipes prove the opposite. In the many years I have known her, she has always cooked delicious food that everyone enjoys—the fact that her dishes are full of healthy goodness are an added bonus, not a complicated hindrance. The pantry list she supplies in this book makes it easy to not be over-whelmed in the grocery store and have on hand all the extra special ingredients I need. I have always turned to Suzanne when I have ques-tions about changing my diet to get more energy and feel better, and now I will turn to this book of recipe gems, knowing that the same care she has taken with me as a friend and healthy living guide she has also taken in sharing her easy, healthy, and delicious recipes. She has taught me that part of being healthy is discovering new foods and rotating my diet because it's so easy to get into a rut and eat the same things every day. This book gave me new ideas about how to reach that goal by showcasing a wide variety of ingredients and preparations. Thank you, Suzanne, for sharing your wisdom!"

—Allison Vander Els,
senior research analyst and mom

"Suzanne's cookbook feels less like a guidebook and more like a conversation with a friend. Suzanne does not preach but rather encour-ages the reader to try various approaches that have worked for her. She has translated her knowledge, experience, creativity, and care for others into delicious, unfussy recipes that nourish the spirit and speak to the uniqueness of all of us. I love healthy food, but when life gets busy and I'm tempted to cut corners, Suzanne reminds us that keeping it simple keeps the peace within our bodies and our minds. I appreciate the complexly flavored but still easy to prepare recipes that stretch my young daughters' taste buds while setting an example of how nurturing and comforting healthy food can be. I want the second half of my life to be as energetic, bold, and fresh as the first—maybe even more so. I needed this book! "

—Leah Jones,
international development consultant and mom

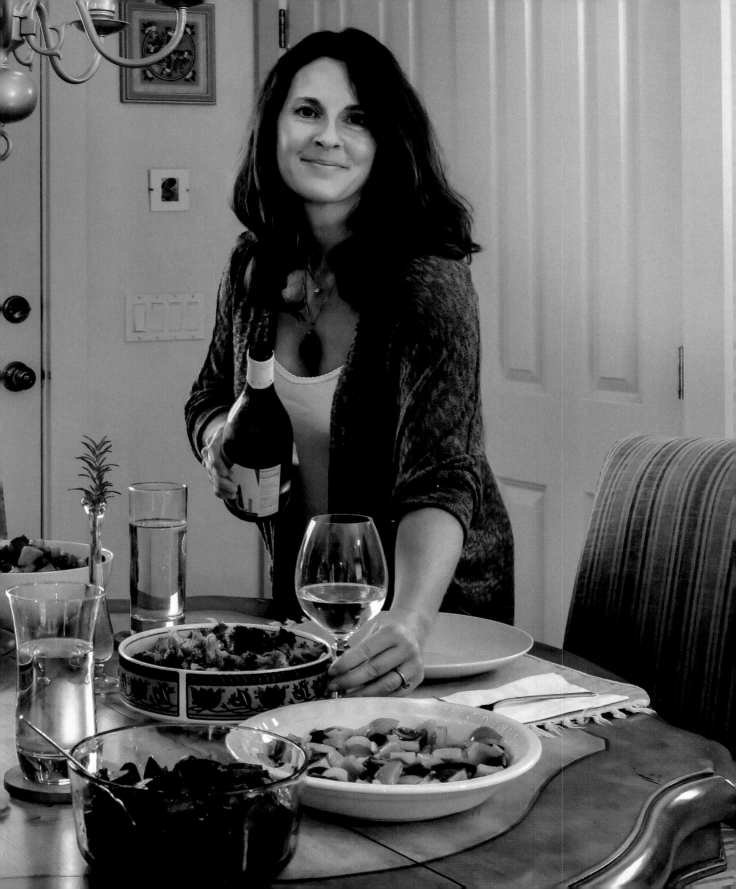

TABLE OF CONTENTS

Acknowledgments...9

INTRODUCTION

About This Book..11

My Story...13

FOOD AND YOUR BODY

Food Rotation...15

Food Intolerance and the Elimination Diet......................16

Food Combining and Digestion......................................18

Salt..19

Sugar...20

Gluten and Wheat..25

Fat and Cholesterol...29

PREPARING YOUR KITCHEN

Quick Tips..33

Essentials for the Pantry...35

Staple Foods, Dried Herbs, and Spices.........................36

Foods to Always Have on Hand 37

My Recipe Guide...40

RECIPES

Fish and Meat..45

Easy Weekend Recipies...73

Vegetable Side Dishes... 81

Hearty Vegetarian Dishes...107

Soups..133

Sauces...141

Salad Dressings...149

Snacks...153

Breakfast 161

Desserts 177

Fun Food and Kitchen Tips..188

Living a Healthy Lifestyle (The Six Foundation Principles)........................190

Resources..194

Index...197

ACKNOWLEDGMENTS

I am grateful to:

My mother, Marie, for providing us with real food when processed food was trendier.

My father, Jack, for instilling in me the love of travel and adventure.

My brother, Michael, for bouncing ideas off in the realm of food.

My daughter, Antonia, for sharing your brilliant ideas and being a fun dinner date since birth.

Mehul, for sharing my love of good food and travel, introducing me to Indian cooking, being my guinea pig, supporting me in the writing of this book, and being a superb partner in this journey of life.

Prafulla Ganatra, for stocking our kitchen with fresh Indian spices.

Faye D'antone and Betty Pijut, for your helpful feedback and encouragement.

Donna Lind, for your artful photography, generosity, fun nature, and encouragement.

Gina Lugo, for generously sharing your vegetable harvest and photos.

Marty Morgan, for generous use of your beautifully hand-crafted pottery.

All my friends, whose excitement for the arrival of this book gave me much inspiration, namely Mary Maestranzi Bourque, Stephen and Allison Vander Els, Jim Saraglow, Jennifer Ware and David Hough, Melissa Montello, and Elena Bergin. Karen Pischke, Nikki Fleenor,

Justine Hardy, Ethel Haddix, and everyone at the Tuesday shares. Sifu Anthony and Sifu Rita Pasquale at United Martial Arts Center.

Everyone whose hard work and creative ideas helped make this book a beautiful reality: Sandra Cook, Donna Lind, Advantage Media Group, Paul Chek, and Antonia Wynn.

Thanks to Turner's Fishery, Common Crow Natural Market, Cape Ann Farmer's Market, Alpirilla Farm, Willow Rest, The Franklin Cape Ann, Duckworth's Bistrot, The Organic Garden, Canaan Farm, and Goose Cove Gardens for providing me with real food.

And special thanks to Marty Adams-DeSimone, Debra Ingalls, Sherry Leavitt, Gina Lugo, and Susan Wharton-Schmitz for good times, having my back, and being my support system.

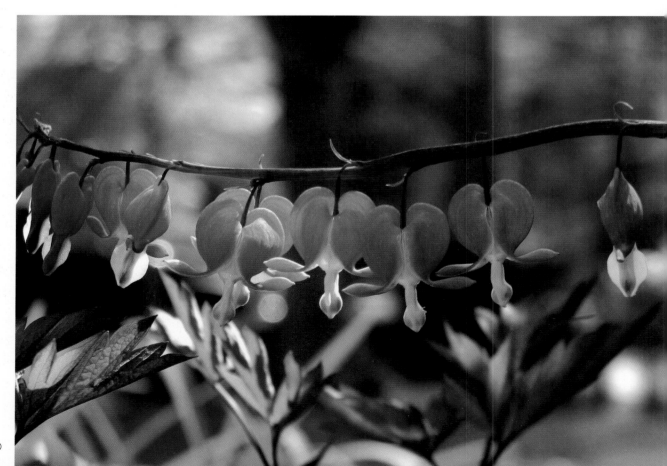

ABOUT THIS BOOK

Welcome to **The Optimal Health Cookbook.** Come on in and enjoy the experience of preparing and eating food that will nourish and delight. Then relish in the healthier you.

The decision to write this book came after seeing how unfamiliar many of my clients were with their kitchens (often due to busy schedules) and how many of them were struggling with food sensitivities. They wanted to prepare healthy meals but didn't think they had the time or know-how. They asked, "What should I be eating, and how do I make it?" This book is the answer.

All of the recipes in this book use fresh, organic ingredients, and most can be prepared and cooked in 30 minutes or less. I've also added a few weekend recipes, which take an hour or more to cook (hands-off) but only minutes to prepare and are worth the wait. I understand that everyone has unique dietary needs. Each recipe is labeled gluten-free (GF), soy-free (SF), nut-free (NF), dairy-free (DF), vegetarian (VG), and suitable for elimination diet (ED), respectively. See pages 16 and 26 for information on elimination diet. It is worth noting that all of the recipes in this book are gluten-free and soy-free and are labeled as such. If you see an asterisk next to a label, it means that the recipe can easily be made to accommodate the referenced dietary need with the substitutions mentioned in the recipe.

I do not subscribe to any particular diet, because everyone's physiology and needs are different. For example, while the Paleo diet may be a better choice than many other diets, its high use of nuts and meat may make it unsuitable for those with a nut allergy and for "carb types" (people who have a higher requirement of carbohydrates at each meal). And a vegetarian diet may be perfect for someone whose body requires a higher amount of carbohydrates but will not serve a "protein type" well. The perfect diet is the one that yields optimal health in your body, mind, and spirit. It's up to you to determine what that diet is, being aware that it may change from time to time as the needs of your body change. In this book you will find plenty of meat and vegetable recipes, and the labels will help determine what is safe and optimal for you to eat.

Cooking is about creativity, nourishment, passion, and love. It's not so much about precision, with exceptions, of course. When trying a new recipe, follow the instructions the first time but add your own flavor to it each subsequent time; a little more of this, a little less of that, or a whole new twist if it suits you. If creating anything in the kitchen sounds daunting, know that with time, practice, and patience, you will learn to cook by intuition rather than by recipe.

The majority of ingredients in this book will be familiar, but I've thrown in some unique ones for fun, variety, flavor, and health benefits. The resource list at the back of this book will help you find unique ingredients and in some cases even the common ones. You can feel confident making all these dishes because they're simple. A great meal does not have to be difficult or complex. These recipes are easy enough for those who don't like to spend much time in the kitchen and creative enough for those who do.

I've included a section with helpful and healthful information and tips, and I invite you to delve in even further by reading some of the books in the resource list. It's your health, after all, and who should look after it if not you? The information and recipes in this book will help give you and your family the nutrition and energy you need. Simply.

May you be inspired and live a long, happy, and healthy life.

Suzanne

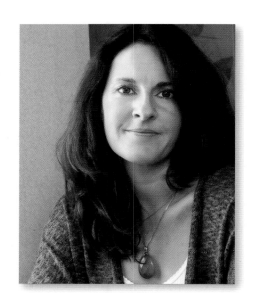

MY STORY

I've always loved to cook and, more so, to eat.

Had I written this book ten years ago, it would have featured as many homemade pasta dishes as I could possibly cook. After learning what many of today's food products, including wheat, can do to a person's body, I decided to embark on a journey to find foods that provide optimal health benefits and taste and are simple to prepare—foods that energize body and mind.

My food journey began with home-cooked meals made by my Italian-American mother. Some of my favorite memories involve making homemade pasta with my mother, grandmother, and great-grandmother and eating stuffed artichokes that my grandmother made especially for me.

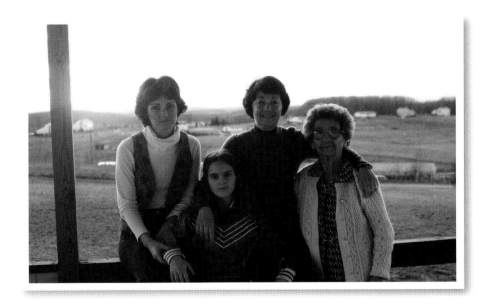

I brought these traditions into my own kitchen and enjoyed creating similar memories with friends and family. These traditions were at risk after choosing to eliminate wheat from my diet, as well as making other dietary changes. While this seemed a sad undertaking at first, I soon became excited to start my own traditions. I knew I would always retain my Italian zest and know-how for good taste, and now I could combine that with optimal health—a perfect pairing. And to add the proverbial cherry on top, somewhere in the midst of this journey I met a beautiful Indian man who, along with his own kitchen-savvy mom, helped impart knowledge and a refined taste for proper Indian food.

While taste and health are crucial parts to a good meal, simplicity is often the deciding factor in whether or not that meal is created in the home kitchen. There are times when I spend hours preparing special meals, but it's what I eat every day that makes or breaks a healthy diet. My goal for this book is to inspire and help you cook delicious, healthy meals at home, even with your busy schedule. I worked for 20 years in the biotech industry while raising my daughter as a single mom. Cooking real food was a priority, and doing it in record time was a must. Let this book help you put good food on your table without going insane!

From my holistic lifestyle studies with the CHEK Institute, informal studies in Ayurveda, participation in countless nutrition seminars, and personal experiences, I have learned and continue to learn how to choose and prepare food to help achieve optimal health. As I incorporate what I've learned, I keep in mind the multitasking involved in juggling family, career, happiness, and health. It is with this amalgam of knowledge and experience, which continues to grow daily, and from my heart, that I write this book, in hopes that it will nourish you and your family in all ways necessary.

FOOD AND YOUR BODY

Food Rotation

Some people love routine and can eat the same thing every day. Others relish trying new foods daily. As with almost everything, there is a happy medium. This happy medium does not come by way of the popular adage *everything in moderation.* The term moderation is subjective, and there are some foods that should not be consumed at all. Food rotation, on the other hand, helps you determine which foods are best for you—in other words, which foods you can easily digest, assimilate, and eliminate. In his book *How to Eat, Move and Be Healthy!*, Paul Chek discusses a four-day food rotation extensively and includes a list of foods based on taxonomy so we can rotate foods that are closely related or in the same family. Using a rotation diet provides our bodies with the opportunity to completely eliminate a particular food (specifically, the protein from that food), giving our bodies a rest before reintroducing it again. Allowing our digestive system to rest in this way will help to identify food intolerances and avoid new ones while giving us the variety of nutrients our bodies need.

The four-day rotation diet consists of eating certain foods during a 24-hour period, then not eating any of those foods again for four days or more. So what you eat on Monday should

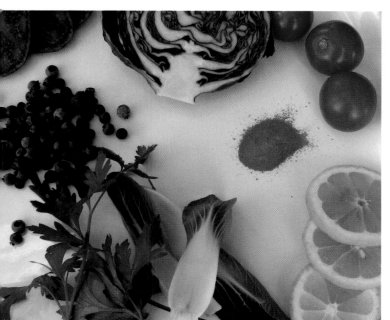

not be eaten again until Friday. Your 24-hour period can begin at breakfast, lunch, or dinner, whatever is easiest on your schedule. Try to abide by the 24-hour rule, but don't stress too much if it occasionally turns into 36 hours.

I recommend using a rotation diet indefinitely, but if you find it too difficult, try using it for a few months to determine food intolerances and detox your system. If you like to eat the same foods every day, the rotation diet will help introduce some variety into your diet, and if you like to change it up so frequently that you stress about what to have for dinner, this will help organize mealtime without becoming boring. It's a win-win plan.

Food Intolerance and the Elimination Diet

Many unpleasant symptoms that we experience in our daily lives can be caused by food intolerance. Food intolerance is the inability to digest or metabolize a food. Most people don't think their lethargy, skin rashes, dry cough, clogged sinuses, achy joints, pain, lack of focus (a.k.a. brain fog), anxiety, or irritability is caused by what they ate for dinner last night or the day before, but, in many cases, it is.

Then there are the symptoms of the digestive tract, such as bloating, gas, cramps, and constipation, which some people may attribute to their food choices. How do we know which food is the culprit? Even healthy, wholesome foods can cause symptoms if you are allergic, intolerant, or sensitive to them. There are medical tests that can be performed to assess your response to certain foods, but they vary in accuracy. An effective, simple, and inexpensive way to figure out which foods may be causing your symptoms is to use an elimination diet. No one knows you better than you, so being aware of how food affects you is the best way to determine whether or not it is a good choice for you. An elimination diet means that you eliminate a list of foods from your diet *completely* for at least one week (two to four weeks if you can), then reintroduce one food at a time, waiting four days before reintroducing the next food. Yes, this does require some time and planning. I've made it significantly easier by providing you with the recipes needed to make it happen, and once you're through you will have a new perspective on life. You'll also wonder how you ever survived day-to-day with those symptoms.

While we are all unique in our physiology and anyone can be allergic, sensitive, or intolerant to just about anything, there are some foods, which I call *heavy hitters* that are believed to cause most of the problems. These are wheat, gluten, soy, dairy, tree nuts, peanuts, eggs, shellfish, corn, sugar, and artificial sweeteners. If you suspect you have a food intolerance, it may also be worth eliminating all grains, nuts, seeds, alcohol, caffeine, foods containing yeast, mushrooms, and nightshades for a period of time (I do not consider these as part of the elimination diet in this book). It's worth noting that oils and fats can sometimes be safely consumed even if sensitivity or intolerance to the protein source exists. For example, many people who don't tolerate dairy can eat butter and ghee with no problems because the protein (often casein or whey) or sugar (often lactose) to which they are intolerant are only present in negligible amounts, if at all, in these fats. This is something you should test under your doctor's recommendation. I've labeled each recipe as gluten-free (GF), soy-free (SF), dairy-free (DF), nut-free (NF), vegetarian (VG), and suitable for elimination diet (ED). I've marked the DF and NF recipes that contain only butter or ghee (and no other dairy) or coconut oil (and no other nuts), respectively, with an asterisk and a note. If you eat dairy-free but can have butter, the DF* recipe is safe for you; likewise if you can have coconut oil but not nuts, the NF* recipes are safe for you. In these recipes I also give alternatives, such as the option of using one oil instead of another in the event that you need to avoid butter or coconut oil. It is also worth noting that many people who are allergic, intolerant, or sensitive to nuts can safely eat coconut. Again, I recommend that you test this with your doctor's approval and supervision.

If you want to delve even deeper into what foods are best for your body, there are several ways to go about getting help. In my practice, I use extensive questionnaires to help you correlate symptoms with their causes, determine your metabolic type (carb, protein, mixed), devise an elimination diet if necessary, and create a diet and lifestyle log to find patterns and identify possible culprits.

Additionally, you can determine your constitution from the perspective of Ayurveda by speaking with an Ayurvedic consultant or filling out a questionnaire online. It simply requires answering some questions about yourself, and then once you've determined your constitution (Vata, Pitta, Kapha, or some combination of the three) you can look at a list of which foods and habits tend to compliment or aggravate that constitution. I've found this information to be quite accurate and that eating and living a lifestyle in line with my constitution helps to keep me balanced. Questionnaires can be found in many books on Ayurveda (see reference section at the back of this book) and online. You can also visit my website EnergizeBodyandMind.com for more information and a short quiz to get you started.

Food Combining and Digestion

Just because you like watermelon and you like eggs doesn't mean you should eat a watermelon omelet. There are certain foods that don't sit well in the stomach if eaten together. For example, in most cases, fruit should be eaten alone, preferably an hour apart from other foods, as it can ferment in the stomach while waiting for the other food to be digested. Different foods require different digestive enzymes and different time frames to digest, so the food waiting to be digested sits in the stomach. While waiting to be digested, fruit can ferment, dairy can curdle, and so on. For example, the stomach acid required to digest melon causes milk to curdle, so you may want to avoid having milk with melon or other sour foods. Poor combinations can produce indigestion, fermentation, putrefaction, and gas formation and, if prolonged, can lead to toxemia and disease.[1] So instead of going for the lobster mac and cheese with pancetta, keep it simple for health.

As usual, there are some guidelines (including avoiding fruit and dairy together), but awareness of how your body reacts to a meal is your best tool. For example, if fruit gives you trouble but not all the time, perhaps it only gives you trouble when eaten with certain other foods. I've known people for whom onions and tomato sauce make for an indigestible combination, but eaten alone, each food is tolerable. Engage your inner scientist and experiment with eating the food alone and with other foods to determine if food combination is the problem.

We often think digestion begins in the stomach. Digestion begins in the mouth and may even begin before that while you're shopping for or preparing your food and your salivary glands are activated. When we put food in our mouths, the tongue sends a message to our brain relaying what it is tasting, so our body can send the appropriate enzymes and acid to our stomach to digest the food. The stomach's job is to break down food particles to a size small enough to enter the small intestine. If the food entering the stomach is too large, it cannot be fully digested and may start to ferment or rot, often causing indigestion. It will also likely be too big for the small intestine to handle properly. Chewing your food slowly and completely, until it's nearly liquid, will make the job of the stomach much easier and will help reduce indigestion and bloating. Chewing slowly and completely is also a great way to connect with the origin and flavors of our food and promote mindfulness.

---

1 Usha Lad and Dr. Vasant Lad, *Ayurvedic Cooking for Self-Healing* (Albuquerque: The Ayurvedic Press, 1994), 45

Salt

The cure for anything is salt water: sweat, tears, or the sea.
—Isak Dinesen

Salt is essential to human life. While many have downplayed the need for salt, it serves the body in a number of key roles.[2]

- Salt is vital to the extraction of excess acidity from the cells of the body, particularly the brain cells.

- Salt aids in balancing blood sugar levels.

- Salt is needed for the absorption of food particles through the intestinal tract.

- Salt clears the lungs of mucus plugs and sticky phlegm, particularly in those suffering from asthma and cystic fibrosis.

- Salt is a strong, natural antihistamine.

- Salt can aid in the prevention of muscle cramps.

- Salt is needed in order to make the structure of the bones firm.

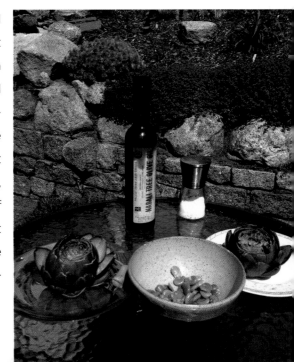

Salt also regulates fluid levels in the body and transmits electrical nerve impulses, not to mention it enhances the taste of food while adding a dimension of its own. Not all salt is created equally. I recommend using unrefined sea salt instead of refined white table salt. New Zealand sea salt is best, as it contains the least mercury. Celtic and French are good, too. Most commercial salt is heavily refined, chemically cleaned, bleached, and treated with anti-caking agents, some of which are aluminum-based. This not only strips the salt of valuable minerals but also makes it difficult for the body to use and eliminate. Iodized salt has been fur-

---

2 Paul Chek, *How to Eat, Move, and be Healthy!* (San Diego: C.H.E.K. Institute, 2004), 77–78

ther processed to chemically bond the iodine with the salt, and dextrose is often added to keep the salt from turning color. Seaweed and seafood are better sources of iodine, an essential nutrient.

Paul Chek states the following in his book *How to Eat, Move and Be Healthy!*:

There are two common sources of salt: land mined and sea salt. Land mined salt from Utah, for example, contains about 98% sodium chloride (NaCl) and the remaining 2% is composed of iron, calcium, and smaller amounts of aluminum and strontium. The sodium from land-locked sources or refined salts hardens and has altered molecular structure. This sodium often remains in the body long after it's done its job, causing joints to swell and kidney problems to develop. Unprocessed sea salt contains about 78% NaCl plus 11% magnesium chloride and smaller amounts of magnesium and calcium carbonate. There are many trace minerals in quality unprocessed sea salt, such as Celtic sea salt, that are beneficial to your body, serving many important regulatory and nutritional functions. Salt consumption, like carbohydrate, protein, and fat consumption, is surrounded with controversy and differing opinions from all sectors of the medical and healthcare community. The medical community generally believes that over-consumption leads to high blood pressure and increased chances of heart disease. Indeed, there are a plethora of studies to suggest this is true. However, most of the research on salt is done on refined salt, not on natural, unprocessed sea salts.

Sugar

Eat less sugar. You're sweet enough already.

I struggled to write about sugar because there is so much to say. Sugar is addictive (emotionally and physically). It affects blood sugar and can lead to a cascade of problems that stem from those spikes and crashes. It feeds bacteria and yeast, and it can cause inflammation, acidity, mucus, hyperactivity, and depressed immune systems. The list goes on.

There is a plethora of data regarding the effects of sugar on the body, and I strongly encourage you to research the subject. The books listed on my resource page are a great place to start. Instead of bombarding you with statistics, I'll focus on a few key points. The amount of sugar in the Standard American Diet (SAD) needs to be vastly reduced in order to achieve optimal health. All refined, processed sugar should be removed (or greatly reduced) from our diet; this includes white sugar, brown sugar, corn syrup, and high fructose corn syrup. The more natural forms of sugar, such as raw honey, maple syrup, coconut palm sugar, molasses, and fruit are still sugar and will affect your blood sugar levels and wreak havoc if overconsumed (overconsumption is approximately >25 grams/day depending on size, metabolic type, and activity level). However, these natural sugars do provide some nutrients and are better options than the refined sugars above. For example, fruit, in its whole form, contains fiber that helps your body eliminate the sugar (a great example of the benefits of eating whole foods). Stevia and xylitol can be used in place of sugar, as they do not affect blood sugar levels the same way sugar does, but each comes with its own set of problems. Stevia is often packaged containing dextrose, sugar alcohols, and natural flavors (a.k.a. chemicals), so you must read the ingredient list on the package (something you should always do anyway) and buy only pure stevia. Most brands of stevia have additives that you don't want, so look carefully (as of this writing, Trader Joe's sells a small bottle of pure stevia). Stevia also has a slight metallic aftertaste, so it may not be to your liking. Xylitol can cause stomach upset in some people and should be used in small quantities. I do not use xylitol in my cooking and baking, and I only use stevia occasionally. I prefer coconut palm sugar and maple syrup (in small quantities). Xylitol and stevia typically do not reduce the body's craving for sweets, so they will not necessarily help curb an addiction to sugar. What about agave?

There's enough controversy surrounding the purity of agave to turn me off, especially since I was never turned on to agave. If you choose to use agave, I recommend doing your due diligence, much like with stevia, and choosing one that is organic and pure. Perhaps you can research some companies to find one whose integrity and values match your own. Please also remember that agave is still sugar, so the quantity used should be limited to avoid repercussions. Cane sugar is a step above processed white sugar but should also be reduced since it is still processed, provides no nutritive value, and does affect blood sugar. If you're questioning whether or not you consume too much sugar each day, read the label on the foods you currently eat (see the list on the next page for alternate names of sugar) and notice how much sugar is added to any given pastry or dessert recipe. With the common morning pastry and latte, most people have exceeded their recommended daily amount of sugar before lunch.

Listen, I have a sweet tooth. Boy, do I ever. When I used to go out to dinner with my friends, and the waiter asked if we wanted to see the dessert menu, my friends all looked at me. I said yes about 80 percent of the time. Back then I also had about an 80 percent chance of catching the flu and all the colds that were going around. Not anymore. Now we all respectfully decline the dessert menu about 80 percent of the time. I do occasionally treat myself to a sweet when dining out, but I'm very discerning.

Over the course of a few months I gradually removed all processed sugar (including cane sugar) from homemade baked goods, including breakfast foods and desserts, with the rare exception (rare being about twice a year, if that). It is important to note the 80/20 rule. This rule states that if you eat and live cleanly 80 percent of the time, you can indulge 20 percent of the time. If you can get to 90/10, that's even better, but 80/20 will suffice. It's important not to replace the stress that a poor diet creates with the stress created by worrying about eating healthy (cleanly) all the time. Enjoy life. This means that if you go out to dinner with your friends Friday night and order dessert, you aren't going to drop dead or be deemed a failure. It means that if you have an occasional day where you just can't find the time or effort to cook clean, organic food, please remember that tomorrow is a new day and you can get back into your healthy groove then. In short, I'm not suggesting you live 100 percent without sweets, unless it suits you. I'm asking you to be aware of your sugar intake, reduce it as much as you can (gradually if necessary), read labels when you purchase food, and switch from re- fined sugar to natural forms of sugar when possible. But now I do have a request that entails 100 percent elimination. Please, for the love of your health, eliminate all artificial sweeteners. ASAP. They are poison. No exaggeration. See the recommended reading at the end of this book for further reading.

After abstaining, or even vastly reducing, sugar and processed food, your tastes will reset. You will have essentially trained your taste buds to prefer food that is less sweet. I've had this experience with both sweet and spicy tastes. I now find most restaurant desserts or pancakes too sweet, and after years of experimenting with Indian spices I'm able to tolerate spicier food than before. In time, you will develop a taste for healthier, real food and you won't want fud[3] or the overload of sugar anymore. You'll appreciate and crave the flavor of real food.

Many people stop craving sugar once they eliminate or reduce it in their diet. For exam- ple, when my clients eliminate gluten from their diet, their sugar cravings tend to decrease

---

3 Fud is a term my friends and I use to describe "fake" food (junk).

or disappear entirely. This is often because they were addicted to bread, pasta, pastries, processed food, and the typical American breakfast foods, all of which quickly convert to sugar (simple carbs) or are laden with sugar. Sugar cravings can indicate addiction, improper macronutrient ratios for your body, fungal infection, emotional eating, and habit, among other things, so if your cravings continue, further exploration may be needed. Those who crave sugar within one to four hours of eating a meal often have the incorrect macronutrient ratio for their body, either too many carbs or too much protein on their plate. Those who hunker down with a box of cookies or a pint of ice cream when they are lonely or depressed are often reaching for something that brings them comfort. And those who go straight for the chocolate (or whatever they fancy) immediately after clearing their dinner plate usually do it out of habit.

These last two examples can often be remedied by remembering what triggered the behavior in the first place and may require you to dig deeper into yourself and your past and perhaps seek help from someone trained in this area. For example, my father went foraging for a sweet every night after dinner while I was growing up, and now when I find myself doing the same, I am aware of what I'm doing and can stop myself (though I choose not to about 20 percent of the time). If you crave healthy food, like fresh vegetables or a healthy source of fat or protein, your body may be telling you that it needs the nutrients in that food. A food craving (even sugar) can indicate a legitimate need, but with sugar that is usually not the case. I invite you to notice the when, what, and where of your cravings (not just sugar) and explore the possible *why* behind them. Knowing why you crave something can help overcome the craving. Always remember to be gentle and patient with yourself during this and all learning processes.

Read labels and look for these names in addition to the word sugar. Many words which end in -ose and -ol are sugars.

Other names for sugar (eliminate or greatly reduce these)

Cane syrup/juice/crystals	Caramel
Corn syrup	Crystalline fructose
Dextrin	Dextrose
D-mannose	Fructose
Fruit juice concentrate	Galactose
Glucose	High fructose corn syrup (HFCS)
Lactose	Maltodextrin
Maltose	Malt syrup (rice, barley)
Rice syrup	Sucanat
Sucrose	Syrup
Treacle	Turbinado
Xylose	

Artificial sweeteners (avoid these)

Alitame	Aspartame
Cyclamate	Equal
Isomalt	NutraSweet
Saccharin	Splenda
Sweet-n-low	Sucralose

Gluten and Wheat

Many people are familiar with the term gluten-free, and quite a few people either know someone who is sensitive to gluten or are sensitive to it themselves. We are coming to realize that gluten-free is not just a fad weight loss diet but that gluten sensitivity or intolerance can cause serious illness. Indeed, a side effect for many who eliminate gluten from their diet is weight loss, but don't you wonder why? Inflammation and toxicity. If you lose weight after eliminating gluten (or any food) from your body, chances are your body was reacting negatively to it. Some scientists, such as neuroscientist Dr. David Perlmutter, believe that virtually everyone is intolerant to gluten to some degree. Even those who don't believe that gluten negatively affects everyone are starting to agree that a growing number of people are sensitive or intolerant to gluten. Unfortunately, the accuracy and relevance of many of the tests used to check for gluten sensitivity is debatable, which does not help in forming a consensus as to the prevalence of gluten disorders.

Gluten, found in grains such as wheat, barley, rye, kamut, and spelt, does not just affect the digestive system in the form of celiac disease, though this is the most commonly recognized disease associated with gluten. Recent studies suggest that gluten intolerance, sensitivity, or allergy may be linked to ADD, ADHD, autism, multiple sclerosis, schizophrenia, Crohn's, rheumatoid arthritis, depression, Graves' disease, Hashimoto's, Alzheimer's, and more. The most common questions I hear regarding this data are, "Why are people suddenly developing intolerance to gluten?" and "Do I have to give up gluten all together, or can I just reduce it?" I will address the first question here and the second a little later in this section.

One theory for why gluten intolerance has become more widespread is that the wheat we are consuming is relatively new. Most of the wheat that we grow in the United States today is different than what we grew 60 years or so ago. Over the course of history, wheat did not evolve much until the twentieth century, when agricultural scientists and governments got involved. With the humanitarian goal of reducing world hunger through increased crop yield and easier harvest, there was seemingly no reason to question the idea of modifying our wheat crop. While the end result made strides in the original goal, very little research was conducted regarding how the new wheat strains would affect long-term human health. Even well before our currently grown strains of wheat were being cultivated, farmers were selectively breeding strains of wheat that produced lighter, fluffier, chewier breads and pastries. It was unknown that an increased amount of gluten proteins in the wheat led to these desirable traits, so how could it be known that increased consumption of these proteins may pose a risk to human health?

I did not jump on the gluten-free bandwagon when I first studied it in 2010. I thought it sounded extreme. But I wanted to know if gluten was something that could be affecting my clients and me. I set out to gather more data and evidence of the connection between gluten and its alleged illnesses. I started reading and learning more about the effects of gluten, and soon my clients were asking me about it. Before recommending that my clients eliminate gluten, I decided to try it myself. My first question was, "Do I have to *completely* eliminate gluten?" The answer is yes. In order to see how you react and feel without gluten (or any particular food substance) in your diet, you have to completely eliminate it. And since it can take days to weeks to completely be out of your system, the most effective test is to eliminate it 100 percent for at least 4–6 weeks to assess how you feel. If you can eliminate wheat in your skin care products also, as our skin absorbs what's on it (this is how things like the nicotine patch work), that would be helpful. These weeks or months of sacrifice may reap incredible health benefits and leave you feeling energized and pain-free. At the very least, you will gain insight into your own body. Elimination diets, especially in conjunction with other lifestyle improvements, have the potential to heal your body, mind, and gut enough to be able to eat the previously offensive food without stress. It will go by very quickly and is totally worth a try. I found it helpful to spend a few weeks weaning myself off gluten and becoming familiar with what I could and could not eat. Once I sorted this out, I began my complete elimination diet. If you choose to go ahead with the elimination diet, give it your full attention and awareness so you don't have to repeat it. Set your goal and stick to it. For more information on conducting an elimination diet, see the section on page 16.

While performing the elimination diet, pay close attention to the symptoms mentioned in the section on food intolerance and elimination diet. Not everyone feels the negative effects of gluten in their digestive system. When I eliminated gluten for my initial 12-week trial period, I didn't have the *wow* experience that many of my clients subsequently had, but I did notice a reduction in joint pain and some weight loss. At the time, I wasn't sure if this was from my gluten-free diet or the fact that I stopped heavy weightlifting, but I remained gluten-free for two years. Then I took a trip to Portugal and decided to indulge in a few pastries. Five days and about as many of Lisbon's famous *pastéis de nata* later, my knees and feet were swollen and in pain, and my jeans were too tight. Within roughly the same time frame, my husband, who was also gluten-free for two years and now indulging in Portugal's finest pastries, became forgetful and a bit foggy in the brain (which became very noticeable as he tried to navigate around a foreign country while I drove).

When people embark on a gluten-free diet, they often ask how they can go gluten-free. The answer is simple but not necessarily easy for some. It may require a change in mind-set about how you shop, prepare, and generally think about food. It may require that you spend a little more money on quality food. Would you rather spend your hard-earned dollars on food that will nourish you and your family or on prescription medications and doctor appointments? Start by buying and eating real, whole, unprocessed food. Meat, vegetables, and fruit are all gluten-free naturally. Eat up!

Figuring out which grains or starches are gluten-free can be confusing. I have included a list for you at the end of this section. It is also useful to check celiac organizations for such information. Eating gluten-free only becomes complicated when processed, packaged, or restaurant food are involved. In these cases we must read all ingredients and ask questions. You'd be amazed at how often wheat flour makes its way into our food supply (condiments, sauces, candy, or fish or meat coated in flour at your favorite restaurant). My best advice is to keep it simple. When in doubt about what you can eat, choose a whole, real, recognizable piece of food.

Many people who switch to a gluten-free diet begin consuming large quantities of ingredients such as guar gum, xanthum gum, potato starch, brown rice flour, etc. I rarely, if ever, use these ingredients, as they can introduce a new set of health concerns if overconsumed. Many packaged gluten-free products and bakery items contain high amounts of sugar—often higher than their gluten-containing counterpart. Eating gluten-free the healthy way requires you to change your mind-set a little. In order to change your life, you have to change your habits, right? In my opinion, eating GF pizza or bread is neither healthy nor tasty, so why do it? You may find a brand of bread, pizza, or other GF counterpart that you like, but beware of the ingredients. You don't want to fill up on sugars, starches, and unrecognizable items. Perhaps you can treat yourself occasionally, but refrain from making it a regular part of your diet.

My goal is not to recreate America's favorite junk foods so that they can be made gluten-free: it is to open your awareness to all the foods that are already GF, naturally. In the following pages, I introduce you and your palate to an array of foods that are natural, healthy, and easy to make.

Gluten-free

Quinoa	Amaranth
Corn	Rice
Oats*	Buckwheat
Sorghum	Teff
Millet	

*naturally gluten-free but are often processed with wheat, so you still need to buy GF oats

Gluten-containing

Wheat**	Barley
Rye	Spelt
Kamut	Farro

**white flour, durham, couscous, bulgar, semolina, triticale, and graham

Look out for wheat (and gluten) in sauces, dressings, gravy, candy, baked goods, processed meat (like lunch meat and hot dogs), self-basting turkey, soy sauce, and seasoned foods (like snacks and rice or pasta in packets).

Fat and Cholesterol

Fat gives things flavor.
—Julia Child

Fat doesn't make you fat. Fat is a nutrient necessary for energy and growth. You need fats to build your body's cell walls, brain cells, and hormones; to insulate nerves; and to carry the fat-soluble vitamins (A, D, E, and K)[4]. Without an adequate amount of healthy dietary fat, your body cannot manufacture hormones or maintain normal cell function, and this slows metabolism. Eating the right amount of healthy fat will help keep you full and slow nutrient absorption so that you'll be able to eat less to maintain energy levels and focus.

So what makes you fat? Food that your body cannot tolerate, subsequently causing inflammation or toxicity, can make you fat. For example, sugar is known for causing inflammation. While glucose, a type of sugar, is necessary for life/energy, fructose, another form of sugar, cannot be utilized by our cells and goes to the liver to be metabolized. If the liver is already overburdened, which many are, the processing of fructose cannot occur, and the fructose is stored as fat. Almost anything that is not utilized or properly processed and eliminated by the body can be stored as fat. For instance, if carbohydrates are not needed or used for energy, they are stored as fat.

Toxins can make you fat. Since our body does not use toxins, it stores any that are unprocessed and eliminated in fat to protect organs from exposure. The more toxins present in your body, the more fat is needed to insulate and protect your organs. Lose the toxins, lose the fat. It's very important not to detox or drop weight too quickly. As you lose fat, the toxins are released, and if your elimination system cannot keep up with the amount of toxins released, the toxins will find something else to bind (somewhere else to go), like your organs or neurological tissue. A safe detox program is one that is gentle and slow and one that will not shock or overburden the organs and elimination system. If you feel the need to detox, I recommend finding someone skilled in detoxification to guide you. Simply improving your diet is sometimes all the detox that is needed.

Animal and vegetable fats are the essential building blocks for cell membrane and hormones. Fat is helpful for nutrient absorption, concentration, hormone regulation and fertility, shiny

4 Laura J. Knoff, NC, *The Whole-Food Guide to Overcoming Irritable Bowel Syndrome* (Oakland: New Harbinger Publications, Inc., 2010), 34

hair, strong nails, and maintaining energy levels. Healthy fats offer the most concentrated source of energy for the body, higher than protein and carbohydrates. Saturated animal fats are hugely beneficial for facilitating healing, enhancing the immune system, and protecting the liver from toxins. They are vital for the transportation of fat-soluble vitamins A, D, E, and K, our anti-aging, free radical-fighting vitamins.

Contrary to popular belief, saturated animal fats are not cholesterol-elevating villains. Elevated cholesterol levels are actually the body's own warning signal, telling us there is a stress being placed on the body. This stress may be from inflammatory foods such as gluten and sugar, pathogenic digestive bugs, or from an emotional stress such as bereavement. Cholesterol actually acts as a precursor for a particular type of hormone (pregnenolone), which helps us deal with stress and helps produce our sex hormones (testosterone, estrogen, and progesterone). Research also shows that it has antioxidant qualities protecting us from free radicals.[5]

It is not possible for humans to eat enough cholesterol-containing foods every day to supply the amount that a human needs. To make up for the difference between what is consumed in the diet and what is needed by our bodies to function properly, our livers and other organs have very active cholesterol synthesis capability (i.e., the capability of manufacturing cholesterol from basic raw material such as carbohydrate, protein, and fat). When there is some cholesterol in the diet, our own synthesis declines, and when there is no cholesterol in our diets (as would be the case with strict vegetarians), the body's cholesterol synthesis is very active. But there is evidence that, for some people, cholesterol is an absolute dietary essential because their own synthesis is not adequate.[6]

There is plenty of literature on trans fatty acids (TFAs), essential fatty acids (EFAs), saturated fats, monounsaturated fats, and polyunsaturated fats. I've listed a few good books in my resources section. For our purposes, it's helpful to know the following basics: Many processed foods, even those touted as healthy, are laden with TFAs. Structurally, TFAs are closer to plastic than fat, and TFA consumption has been linked to heart disease and elevated cholesterol levels.[7] According to the CDC (Centers for Disease Control and Prevention), the major contributors to Americans' overconsumption of artificial TFAs include

5 Karen Maidment, *Meals That Heal* (Karen Maidment; first edition December 15, 2012)
6 Mary G. Enig, Ph.D, *Know Your Fats: The Complete Primer for Understanding the Nutrition of Fats, Oils, and Cholesterol* (Silver Spring: Bethesda Press, 2000), 50
7 Paul Chek, *How to Eat, Move, and be Healthy!* (San Diego: C.H.E.K. Institute, 2004), 72

fried food, snacks like microwave popcorn, frozen pizzas, cake, cookies, pie, margarines and spreads, ready-to-use frosting, and coffee creamers.

EFAs are fats (polyunsaturated) that our bodies need but cannot make and must be included in our diet. The omega-6 EFAs can be found in grains, meat, and most vegetable oils, including sunflower, corn, and safflower. The omega-3 EFAs are found in leafy greens, oily fish, flax seeds, chia seeds, walnuts, eggs, and to a lesser degree in animal meat. Our bodies need the proper ratio of omega-6 to omega-3, and because of the foods we eat and the way they are manufactured, Americans tend to be too high in omega-6, throwing off this ratio. This is why so many people are finding ways to get more omega-3 EFAs in their diet.

I've included a list of saturated, monounsaturated, and polyunsaturated fats so you know where to begin. Saturated fats can be found in animal fat (including lard, ghee, and butter), coconut (and its oil), and palm oil. These oils keep well and are the best oils for cooking as they do not tend to go rancid even when heated.

Monounsaturated fats are usually liquid at room temperature and keep well (though not as long as saturated fats). These oils can be used for cooking at moderate temperatures, such as light sautéing and baking up to 325°F /163°C. Examples of oils which are high in monounsaturated fat are olive oil, avocado oil, and peanut oil.

Polyunsaturated fats are liquid at room temperature and often remain liquid even in the refrigerator. These fats oxidize (go rancid) very easily when exposed to heat, light, and oxygen. This means that these oils don't keep long, so buying small bottles, storing in a refrigerator or cabinet, and keeping the lid on tight will help. Examples of polyunsaturated oils are most vegetable oils, including corn, safflower, sunflower, soybean, and sesame, as well as flax and fish oil.

The amount of dietary fats needed varies from person to person, but some amount of healthy fat should be consumed at every meal. If you are not in the habit of eating fats and have been following a low-fat diet for a long period of time, add good quality fats into your diet gradually.

Some examples of good fats are (all fats should be organic) butter, ghee, coconut oil, cold-pressed extra-virgin olive oil, nuts, avocado, fat from pasture-raised animals, flax seeds, chia seeds, and hemp seeds. Fats that should be avoided are trans fats, hydrogenated oils, most fats and oils found in processed food and chips, oil that is old and stale as it has likely oxidized, unsaturated oil which has been heated to high temperature (most fried foods), margarine, and fat substitutes.

In the words of Julia Child, who seemed to appreciate the worth of fat,

"Bon appétit!"

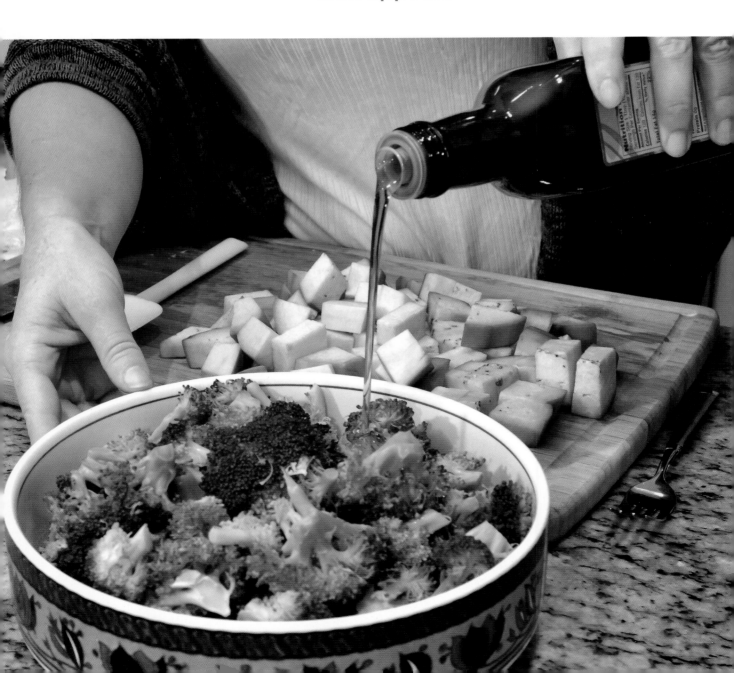

PREPARING YOUR KITCHEN

Quick Tips

Preparing real food fresh every day is the best way to achieve optimal health through diet. However, if you don't have time for this, and grocery shopping and cooking become a source of stress, you are negating your effort to move toward health. If you can grocery shop two to three times per week and cook almost daily, do it. If not, here are some tips to experiment with to see if they alleviate your time crunch. Once many fruits and vegetables are chopped, they begin to oxidize and lose freshness, potency, and sometimes nutrients, so try to minimize chopping too far ahead of time (same-day washing and chopping is best).

1. Multitask while prepping and cooking. For example, if a recipe calls for a pot of boiling water, put it on the stove before you begin chopping vegetables. Also, prep what needs to go in the pan first, and then prep the remaining ingredients while the first ones sauté. I've outlined these tips in the preparation section of each recipe, so reading the prep steps before you begin will help. Sometimes it's best to prep everything before you begin, and sometimes you can prep while cooking. Experiment—you'll get better with practice.

2. Not only can you prep ingredients within a dish while part of it is cooking, in many cases you can prep your side dish while the main dish is cooking. Choose your protein and vegetable dishes, and then read the preparation steps for each dish before you begin. If either dish cooks for 15 minutes or more, you can get that in the oven (or on the stove) first and then begin the other, quicker dish.

3. Steamed vegetables such as green beans, broccoli, and asparagus can be a quick side dish for any main meal. Steam, then drizzle with extra virgin olive oil, salt, and pepper, and you're done. This is the fastest, easiest way to get nutritious food on the table, and you can have a different vegetable every day. Add a little garlic, herbs, spices, or ginger while it's steaming, now and then, for more variation, and

try shopping at a different grocery store for more options. Whole Foods has a fantastic variety of produce. Buy three different vegetables while you're shopping, and you have an easy vegetable dish for half your week.

4. Try using a Crock-Pot for meats and stews and a pressure cooker for rice or vegetables that take longer to cook, like whole artichokes. Be careful to follow instructions when using these pieces of equipment.

5. If there is time, clean the dishes/utensils you are done with while things are cooking.

6. Keep a shopping list going at all times. When you're running low on something, add it to the list so you're ready when it comes time to shop. I use the notes app on my phone.

7. Be creative, go easy on yourself, and have fun. Put on some music if you like. Set your intention and focus on the task at hand. Cooking is a great way to practice being in the present moment. If it doesn't come out perfect the first time, try it again, tweaking as you like. You won't mind the time used for cooking if you're enjoying yourself. Cooking with love and good intentions always makes the food taste better. Really.

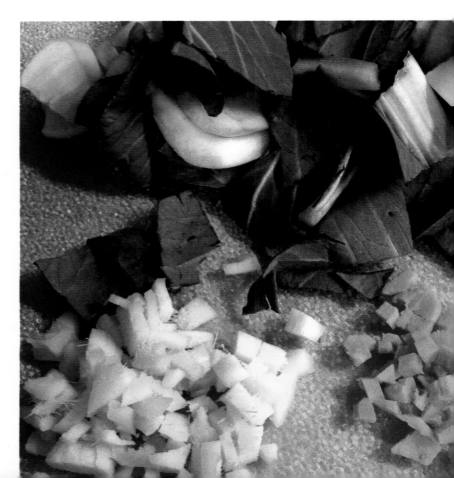

Essentials for the Pantry

Accessories

- Small chopper (found in most grocery stores, hardware stores, department stores, and online, and costs around $25)

- Sharp knife (owning a quality knife is half the battle—getting it professionally sharpened regularly is the other half and will speed prep time)

- Wooden or silicone spoons and spatulas

- Large cutting board, preferably bamboo or other wood (plastic retains bacteria, glass dulls knives but cleans easily in the dishwasher)

- Blender or Vitamix® (a Nutribullet® also works for smaller portions and is less expensive)

- Glass, stainless steel, and/or cast iron pots and pans (avoid nonstick pans which can leach perfluorooctanoic acid—PFOA—into your food)

- Glass storage containers (such as Pyrex® and CorningWare®)

- Stainless steel or glass measuring cups and spoons

- Vegetable steamer—either a pot with a steamer included or a silicone or stainless steel one found at most grocery stores

- Salad spinner

- Strainer (and a colander)

- Citrus reamer (preferably glass or ceramic)

- Garlic press (stainless steel)

- Coffee grinder—this isn't an essential, but it does come in handy for freshly grinding spices, seeds (such as sesame or flax), and coffee beans.

Staple Foods, Dried Herbs, and Spices

Having the following foods and spices on hand allows me to quickly throw a meal together anytime:

Herbs and Spices

- Sea salt

- Black pepper

- Crushed red pepper

- Cinnamon (ground and sticks)

- Cayenne pepper

- Paprika

- Cumin
  (I keep both seeds and powder)

- Coriander powder

- Ground ginger

- Turmeric powder

- Herbs de Provence

- Oregano

- Rosemary

- Thyme

- Bay leaves

- Mustard (ingredients should be limited to mustard seed, water, cider vinegar, and sea salt)

Additionally, I keep fennel powder and seeds, fenugreek, cloves, cardamom, nutmeg, lavender, curry leaves, saffron, dhana jiru (a mix of cumin and coriander), and dulse granules.

Foods to Always Have on Hand
(as long as you and your digestive system like them)

- Fresh lemons and/or limes (not the stuff in the bottle)

- Fresh ginger

- Fresh garlic

- Organic butter (Salted and unsalted. I also use organic ghee occasionally.)

- Organic extra-virgin olive oil (stored in a dark place like a cabinet instead of on your counter)

- Organic virgin coconut oil (stored in a dark place like a cabinet)

- Vinegars (apple cider, balsamic, red wine, and coconut)

- Eggs

- Avocados

- Salad greens/leafy greens (variety!)

- Fresh and frozen vegetables (fresh as often as possible, especially in season)

- Pumpkin purée (BPA-free cans or tetra packs)

- Nuts and nut butters* (almond, cashew, walnut, pecan, and coconut)

- Sesame seeds, raw (you can toast them as needed—they'll retain freshness this way)

- Fruit, seasonal fresh and frozen

- Quinoa

- Rice

- Sprouted mung beans (trüRoots is a good brand) and other lentils

- Mung bean, black bean, or buckwheat pasta

- Creamy buckwheat or GF oats

- Jar of high-quality olives, such as Kalamata

- Jar of capers (not a must, but it can add lots of flavor in a pinch)

- Canned sardines in water (one of the few quality meat/fish sources one can have on hand)

- Organic broth (chicken, vegetable, beef, and mushroom)

- Jar of pure crushed tomatoes or tomato sauce (read labels!)

Note: I recommend eating the rice and pastas listed above no more than once per week. I keep them handy for days when I don't have time to shop and need to find a meal from what's in my pantry.

Flours

- Coconut flour

- Oat flour (gluten-free)

- Almond flour or meal

- Chestnut flour

- Sorghum flour, millet flour, and/or buckwheat flour

*Storage note: It is best to buy nut meals and flours in small batches to ensure freshness. I store most of my flour in the refrigerator and my nut flour/meal in the freezer, as it can go rancid rather quickly. I also keep nuts in the refrigerator and consume them within a month or so. Lately, I've been making my own nut meal, as needed, using my Vitamix. It's fresher and cheaper.

Sweetness

- Maple syrup and maple sugar

- Honey (raw and local if possible; the cloudier, the better)

- Coconut palm sugar

- Stevia (only if it's pure stevia—watch out for stevia mixed with maltodextrin and other stuff)

- Pure vanilla

- High-quality cacao powder, nibs, and dark chocolate—the darker the better!

My Recipe Guide

Assume everything in my ingredient list is organic. Rather than continuously specifying organic basil for example, I simply write basil. I buy organic whenever possible. This includes fruits, veggies, meat, dairy, eggs, grains, legumes, spices, oils, and chocolate, so assume that all of my ingredients are organic even though it's not specified for each item.

Since buying organic isn't always possible due to availability and cost (though I often forgo buying something if it isn't organic), here is a list of foods that are more vital to buy organic (typically due to heavy pesticide use). Any food that tends to be genetically modified (GMO), such as corn and soy products, should also be organic (as of this writing, the organic label certifies that the product is non-GMO).

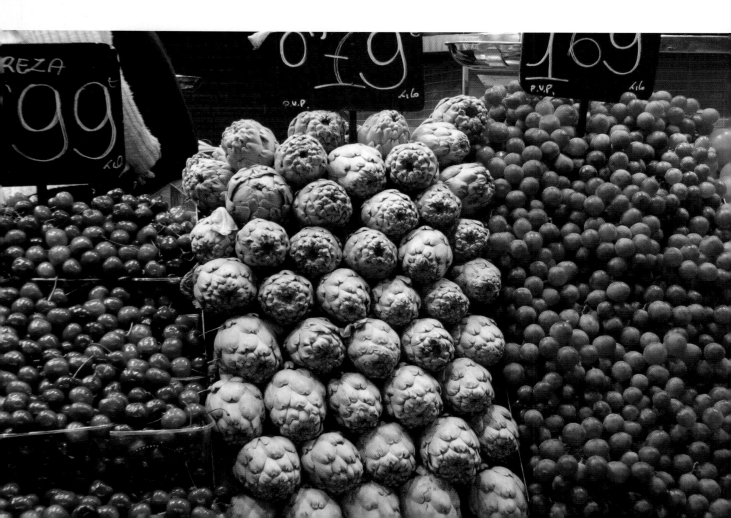

Apples	Fruit juices	Strawberries	Eggs
Pears	Dried fruits	Spinach	Oils
Cherries	Apricots	Celery	Corn
Grapes	Lemons	Bell peppers	Soy
Raisins	Limes	Potatoes	Coffee
Peaches	Raspberries	Milk/cream	Nuts
Nectarines	Blueberries	Butter	Meats

Why buy organic? Organic foods are grown in nutrient-rich soil (made so by farming techniques like crop rotation) without the use of toxic, synthetic pesticides, herbicides, fungicides, or chemical fertilizers. Many studies suggest that utilizing nutrient-rich soil yields food higher in nutrients. Makes sense to me. It is also thought that organic food contains a higher amount of energy (is more alive) than conventional food. Organic foods are also non-GMO (not genetically modified), are better for the environment, and help support many small, local farmers.

For more on organic versus conventional food, you can read *How to Eat, Move and Be Healthy!* by Paul Chek and do a search for Virginia Worthington (she published a study comparing the two). There are many studies on both sides of the argument, and I encourage you to research the subject on your own, paying close attention to who conducted, published, and funded any particular study to be sure there was no conflict of interest.

You can also assume everything in my ingredient list is washed. I always wash my fruits and vegetables, even if they are organic, right before eating or cooking them. I have a water filter under my kitchen sink ($25–$30 at Amazon), so the water that I wash and cook my food in is free of as many contaminants as possible. I spin the washed food in a salad spinner when appropriate, so it won't taste watery, especially if I'm eating it raw.

The ingredient list for each recipe is formatted so that you can easily use it as a shopping list. Simply check off the staples you already have, and enjoy choosing the remaining fresh ingredients for your delicious meal.

Abbreviations

EVOO = extra-virgin olive oil

S&P = salt and pepper to taste; start with 1/2 tsp. of each and increase from there.

GF = gluten-free

DF = dairy-free

NF = nut-free

VG = vegetarian (not vegan)

SF = soy-free

ED = suitable to eat during elimination diet

tsp. = teaspoon

TBSP = tablespoon

~= I often don't bother measuring—I just approximate. This comes with experience. Use measurements as a guideline, and then adjust according to your taste. It's also worth noting that cooking times will vary with different ovens, so you may need to experiment with the times I've written.

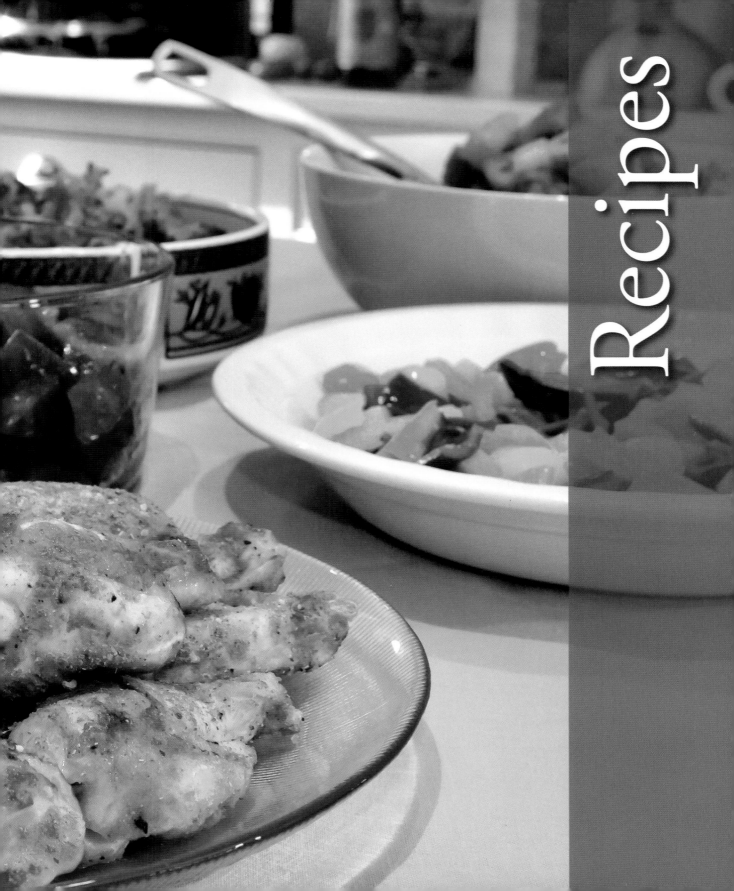

Recipes

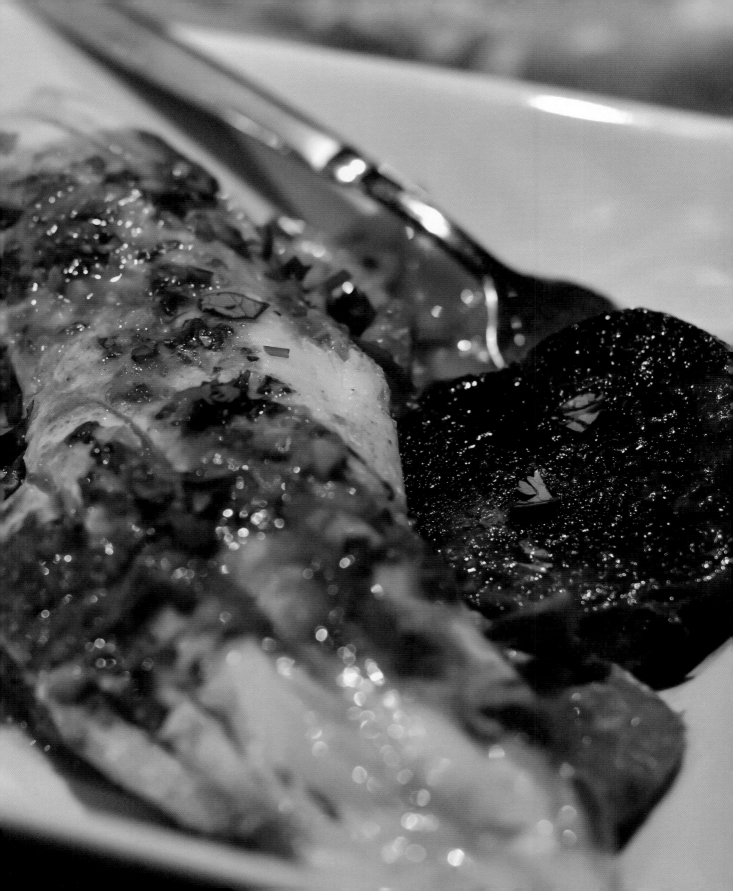

FISH

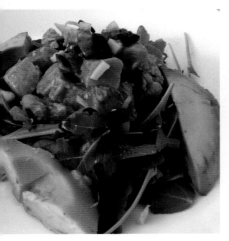 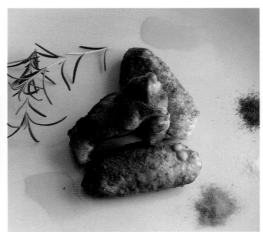 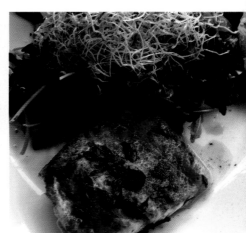

& MEAT

TUNA STEAKS

(GF, SF, DF, NF, ED)

Prep time: 10 minutes

Cook time: 5–10 minutes

Serves 2

Ingredients

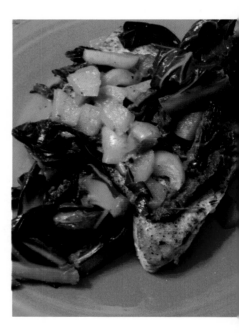

2 tuna steaks (3/4–1 inch thick or your preference)*

2-inch piece of fresh ginger, peeled and chopped

Sesame oil (can use coconut oil if preferred, but it will not be strictly nut-free)

Salt and pepper to taste

Sesame seeds

1/2 teaspoon coriander powder or *dhana jiru*** (optional)

Hot sesame oil (optional)

Kelp flakes (optional)

Preparation

1. Press sesame seeds and S&P onto raw steaks. Put a small amount of oil in a skillet over medium heat. When skillet is hot, add the coriander and half the ginger and sauté for about a minute.

2. Add tuna steaks and cook for about two minutes on each side. For best taste, tuna should be rare. Serve with remaining raw ginger and hot sesame oil if desired.

*Start with fresh, sushi-grade tuna from a reputable source, preferably a local fish market. Buy steaks as thick as you want (I like mine ~3/4-inch, but most people prefer them thicker). Due to the possibility of tuna (and other large fish) being contaminated with mercury, I recommend eating it no more than once every two weeks.

***Dhana jiru* is a combination of cumin and coriander widely used in Indian cooking.

· ·

Serving Suggestion: Serve with sautéed greens and peppers or with steamed vegetables.

· ·

HAKE WITH CHIMICHURRI

(GF, SF, DF, NF, ED)

Total prep/cook time: 15 minutes

Serves 4

Ingredients

2 pounds fresh hake filets
(can also use haddock, cod, or other similar white fish)

For the chimichurri

1 packed cup of fresh cilantro

1/2 packed cup fresh parsley

2 cloves of garlic

1 teaspoon crushed red pepper flakes

1 teaspoon oregano

3 tablespoons red wine vinegar (can use lemon juice instead if you prefer)

1/3 cup EVOO

Salt and pepper to taste

Preparation

1. Preheat oven to 300°F. Bake fish for 15 minutes per inch of thickness.

2. While fish is cooking, add chimichurri ingredients, except S&P, to a chopper or blender, and gently blend until mixed. Stir or blend in S&P to taste.

3. When done, remove fish from oven and place on serving dish. Drizzle with chimichurri sauce.

Note: The chimichurri sauce can be made up to one day ahead and refrigerated. Pesto also goes well on white fish. See pesto recipe on page 143.

HADDOCK AND VEGETABLES IN FOIL

(GF, SF, DF, NF, ED)

Prep time: 15 minutes

Cook time: 20 minutes

Serves 4

Ingredients

2 pounds fresh haddock, skinned

2 carrots, outer layer peeled

1 box (5 ounces) baby spinach or other leafy green (such as chard or kale)

1/2 box of cherry tomatoes, sliced in half (or chopped regular tomatoes)

Juice of 1 lemon

1 tablespoon fresh oregano (can also use dried)

Salt and pepper to taste

A sprinkling of dulse granules (optional)

Preparation

1. Preheat oven to 325°F, or heat up the grill. Chop tomatoes.

2. Place fish in a large piece of heavy-duty foil. I usually line the foil with parchment paper as well, but this is not necessary. Pour 3/4 of the lemon juice on the fish. Sprinkle with dulse (if desired), 1/2 TBSP oregano, salt, and pepper.

3. Using a potato peeler, peel the carrots directly on top of the fish (let the shavings fall on top of the fish).** Put spinach and tomatoes on top of carrots, sprinkling remaining oregano as you go. Add the remaining lemon juice and more S&P to taste.

4. Wrap the foil loosely but securely. Place on grill for 15–20 minutes or in the oven for 15–20 minutes or until fish is fully cooked.

5. Open foil carefully, as steam may burn. Do not overcook fish. If carrots are a little crunchy but fish is done, your meal is ready! The second-best part of this meal is the easy clean up.

** You can also use a cheese grater for the carrots and add the shavings to the fish.

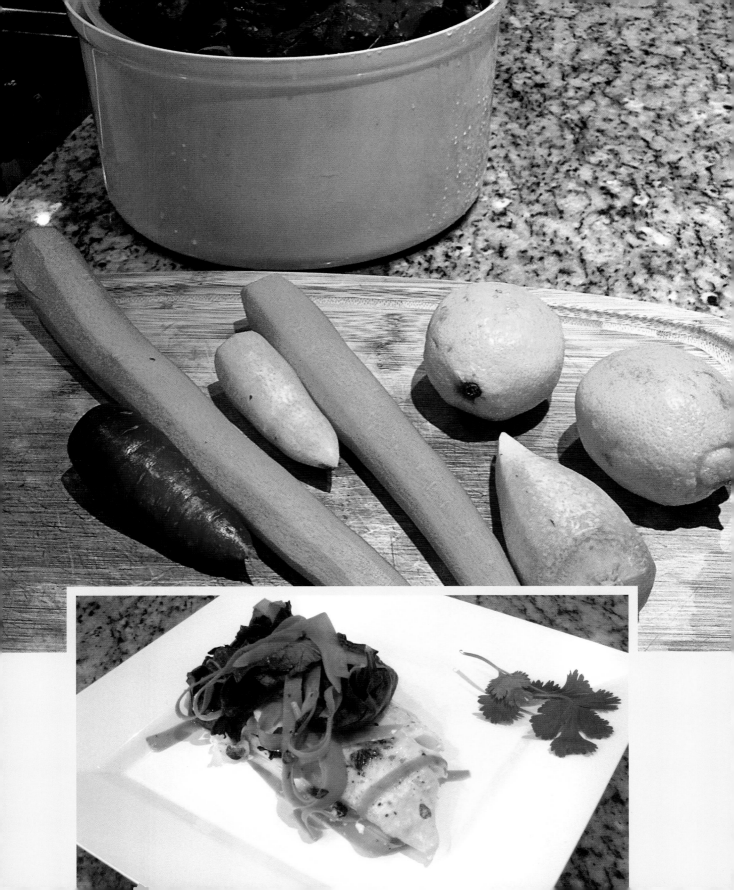

HADDOCK WITH FRESH SALSA

(GF, SF, DF, NF, ED)

Prep time: 15 minutes

Cook time: 15 minutes

Serves 4

> Freshness emanates from this dish, and it's so simple. Put fish in the oven, and then mix cherry tomatoes, onion, parsley, and S&P in a chopper—boom, done.

Ingredients

2 pounds fresh haddock filets, skinned

Pinch of dulse granules (optional)

Fresh tomatoes (3–4 large, 8 small or medium, or 1 package of cherry tomatoes)

1/2 bunch of parsley (can also use cilantro)

1/2 red onion (optional)

1/2–1 jalapeño or shishito pepper with seeds removed (optional)

1–2 teaspoons capers (start with 1 tsp. and add more to taste)

Salt and pepper to taste (if using capers, you may not need salt; if using a jalapeño or shishito pepper, you may not need black pepper)

Preparation

1. Preheat oven to 300°F. Place fish in ovenproof dish, sprinkle lightly with dulse if desired, and bake for 15 minutes per inch of thickness (~12–15 min). Do not overcook.

2. While fish is cooking, roughly chop tomatoes, onion, and pepper, and blend in a chopper or blender with remaining ingredients.

3. Plate the fish and top with tomato salsa.

. . . .

Serving Suggestion: Serve with kelp noodles (see recipe on page 111) and a simple green salad.

. . . .

FISH FILETS WITH OLIVE TAPENADE AND LEMON

(GF, SF, DF, NF, ED)

Prep time: 5 minutes

Cook time: 15 minutes

Serves 4

Ingredients

2 pounds fresh fish filet

(striped bass, haddock, cod, hake, tilapia, salmon, char, or similar)

1 jar (~4 oz.) of olive tapenade (I use organic Divina brand, or you can grind your own Kalamata olives and capers using a chopper, blender, or mortar and pestle.)

Black pepper to taste

2 teaspoons oregano (fresh or dried) or herbs de Provence

1 lemon

Preparation

1. Preheat oven to 300°F.

2. Place fish in a glass, oven-proof dish and sprinkle with pepper. Place in oven and cook 15 minutes per inch of thickness (which will be about 15 minutes for most filets). Do not overcook.

3. If making your own tapenade, prepare it while fish is cooking by adding olives, capers, and pepper to a chopper, blender, or mortar and pestle. Mix until well blended and chopped.

4. Once fish is done, spread tapenade over fish in a thin layer. You can always add more if you desire, but tapenade can be salty and strongly flavored, so add it little by little. Top with a bit of oregano and freshly squeezed lemon, which helps cut the saltiness of the tapenade.

Note: Prepare your favorite vegetable dish while fish is cooking.

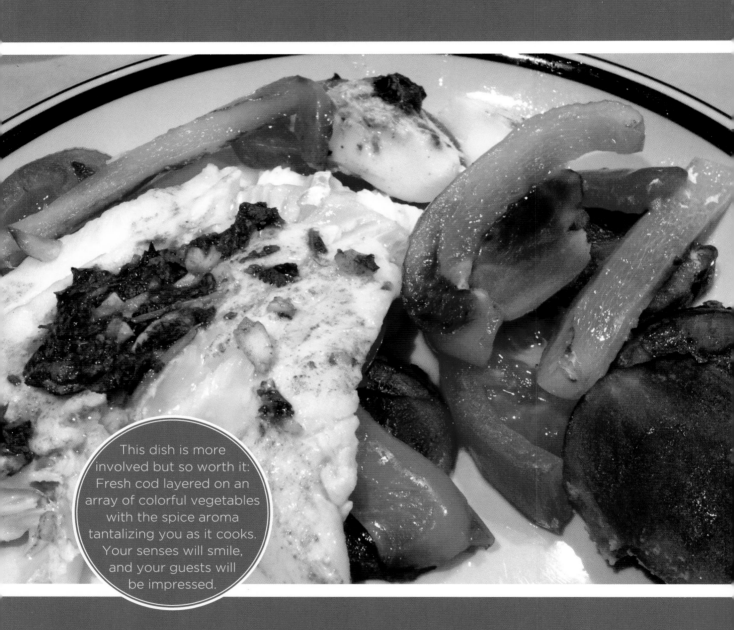

This dish is more involved but so worth it: Fresh cod layered on an array of colorful vegetables with the spice aroma tantalizing you as it cooks. Your senses will smile, and your guests will be impressed.

COD WITH MOROCCAN SPICES

(GF, SF, DF, NF, ED)

Prep time: 45 minutes

Cook time: 30 minutes

Serves 4

Ingredients

For fish and vegetables

2 pounds cod or haddock fillets, skinned and cut into 6 pieces

1 pound small–medium potatoes (Use purple ones if you can find them; they add great color.)

2 tablespoons olive oil (can also do without)

2 bell peppers (preferably yellow or orange)

2 medium tomatoes

2 tablespoons fresh lemon juice

For sauce

1 cup fresh cilantro (can also use flat-leaf parsley or a combination of cilantro and parsley)

5 garlic cloves

1/3 cup fresh lemon juice

2 teaspoons paprika

1 1/2 teaspoon salt

1 1/2 teaspoons ground cumin

1/4 teaspoon cayenne

1/4 cup olive oil

Preparation

1. Preheat oven to 375°F. Slice peppers into 1/4-inch-wide strips.

2. Prick each potato once with a fork, then rub potatoes with 1/2 tablespoon of oil. Place potatoes on a baking pan or sheet, and bake until just tender

or for about 30 minutes (proceed to next steps while potatoes cook). Once potatoes are tender, cool to room temperature, and cut crosswise into 1/4-inch-thick slices. If you use larger potatoes, slice in half or quarters before baking for equivalent cooking time. After you remove potatoes from the oven, lower the oven temperature to 350°F.

3. While potatoes are cooking, heat 1 1/2 tablespoons of oil in a heavy skillet over medium heat, then add bell peppers and sauté, stirring occasionally, until just tender, for about 12 minutes.

4. While peppers and potatoes are cooking, slice tomatoes, remove large stems from the cilantro, and peel the garlic. Purée all sauce ingredients except oil in a chopper, food processor, or blender. With motor running, add oil in a slow stream.

5. Spread potato slices evenly in a 13 x 9 x 2-inch glass baking dish, and season with S&P. Top with peppers, then tomatoes and fish, seasoning each layer with S&P to taste. Sprinkle fish with 2 TBSP lemon juice.

6. Pour sauce evenly over fish, and bake in the middle of oven at 350°F until fish is just cooked through or for about 20–25 minutes. The fish is done when a piece easily flakes off with a fork but there is still a slight sheen to it.

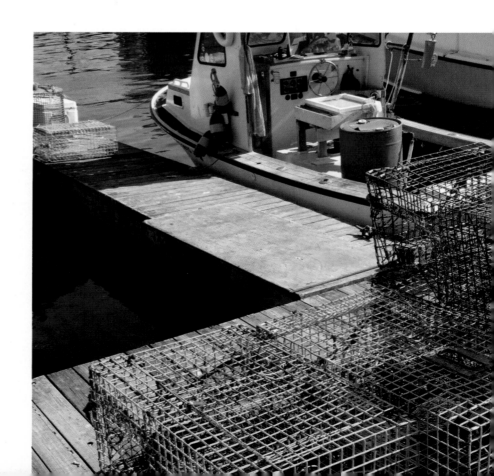

ARCTIC CHAR WITH CAPERS AND DILL

(GF, SF, DF, NF, ED)

Prep time: 5 minutes

Cook time: 15 minutes

Serves 2

Ingredients

- 1 pound Arctic char (can also use salmon)
- 2–3 tablespoons capers
- 2–3 tablespoons fresh or dried dill (enough to lightly cover fish)

Preparation

1. Preheat oven to 300°F.

2. Place fish in a glass oven-proof dish, and cover with capers and dill.

3. Place fish in oven, and cook 15 minutes per inch of thickness. Do not overcook.

Note: Prepare vegetable dish while fish is cooking.

. . . .

Serving Suggestion:
Serve with broccoli,
stuffed artichoke or
artichoke hearts.

. . . .

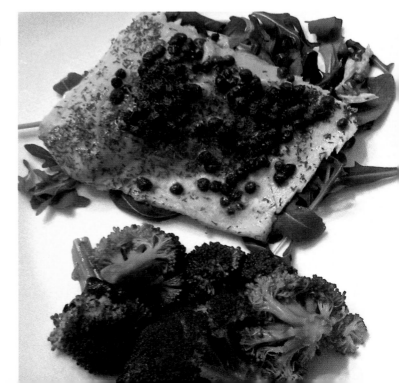

NEW MOON SALMON (VERY BLACKENED SALMON)

(GF, SF, DF, NF, ED)

Prep time: 5 minutes

Cook time: 8–10 minutes

Serves 2–3

Ingredients

- 1 pound filet of fresh, wild salmon with the skin on (or farm-raised if from a reputable source)
- 1 tablespoon paprika
- 2 teaspoons cayenne pepper (or powdered red chili)
- 1/2 teaspoon salt
- 2 teaspoons oregano (fresh or dried)
- 1 teaspoon thyme, rosemary, or herbs de Provence
- 2–3 tablespoons of your favorite high-heat-tolerant oil (coconut oil or avocado oil, for example)
- 1 teaspoon ancho chili powder (optional)

Preparation

1. Mix herbs and spices in a small bowl. Coat the flesh side of the fish with the herb/spice mix.

2. Heat oil in a heavy-bottomed pan (stainless steel or cast iron) on medium-high heat until it almost begins to smoke (about one to two minutes). Add fish to the pan, spiced-flesh side down, and immediately reduce heat to a simmer. If any spice mixture remains, you can sprinkle it on the skin side now.

3. Cook for two to three minutes, and then flip and cook another five to six minutes. These cooking times are for a filet about an inch thick. Adjust cooking time accordingly for a thinner or thicker filet. Lean toward the lower cooking times. Do not overcook. Salmon is best served rare.

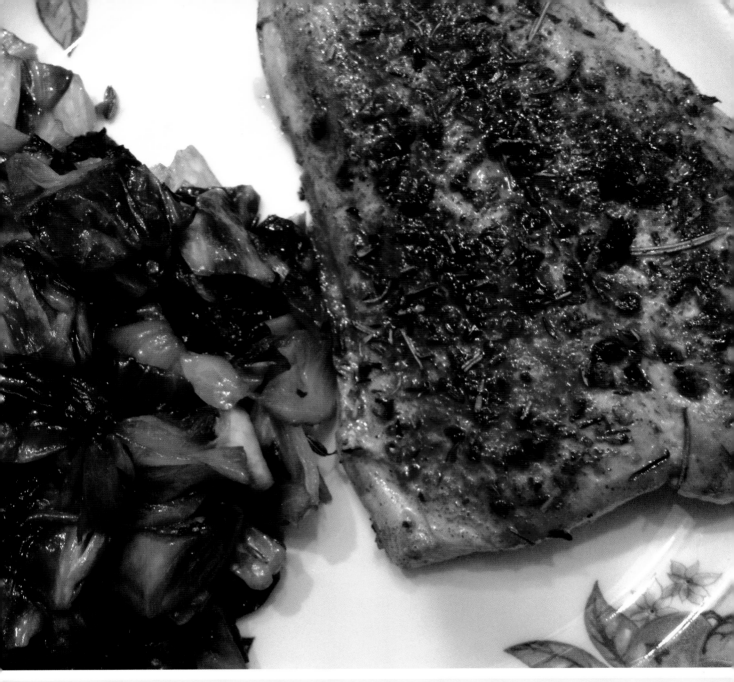

Salmon served with radicchio with fennel (recipe on page 95).

I was not a salmon lover until I tried this recipe. If you enjoy the taste of salmon and don't enjoy a lot of spice, I recommend using less herbs and spices than I have listed here (try half). If you don't enjoy the strong taste of salmon, try this recipe, tweaking the amount of spice to your liking, and you may become a salmon lover.

RED FISH WITH ROASTED RADICCHIO AND SPINACH

(GF, SF, DF, NF, ED)

Prep time: 10 minutes

Cook time: 10 minutes

Serves 2

Ingredients

1 pound red fish filets (sole, flounder, or similar can also be used)

1 head of radicchio

1 box (5 oz.) of organic baby spinach

1 teaspoon dried oregano, plus more to taste

Crushed red pepper to taste

EVOO

Salt to taste

Preparation

1. Preheat oven to low broil.

2. Wash radicchio, then spin dry and chop into ~2–3 inch pieces.

3. Place radicchio into rectangular glass pan, and toss with EVOO, oregano, crushed red pepper (1/2 tsp.), and salt.

4. Lay the pieces of fish out, and sprinkle one side with crushed red pepper, salt, and oregano. Pour ~2 TBSP EVOO into a frying pan, and then turn on medium heat.

5. Place radicchio under the broiler without being too close to the broiler (rack in usual middle spot). Cook ~six minutes or until just brown.

6. While the radicchio is cooking, place fish, herbed side down, into heated frying pan. Now sprinkle the remaining side with crushed red pepper, salt, and oregano. Cook for about two minutes, and then turn the heat to low-medium and flip fish. Cook for another three to four minutes.

7. When the radicchio is just starting to brown on the tips, add the spinach right on top of it (no need to mix). I literally just open the oven, pull the pan out a bit, and throw the spinach right on top without fully removing the pan. It should take about ten seconds! Continue to cook another minute.

8. Remove radicchio and spinach from the oven, and gently stir in the spinach. The spinach will cook as it mixes with the warm radicchio.

9. Serve the fish and radicchio and spinach as soon as they come out of the oven. A glass of crisp white wine sure sounds good right about now... Enjoy!

Alternate preparation for red fish with radicchio and spinach:

Same ingredients, plus fresh guacamole (see page 159 for homemade guacamole recipe).

1. Add 1 TBSP coconut oil (can also use EVOO) to a frying pan, and place on medium-low heat.

2. Add radicchio and herbs/spices, and sauté two to three minutes until just starting to brown.

3. Add spinach and sauté another two minutes or until just soft and wilted. Place in serving bowl (or plate into individual dishes) and set aside.

4. Using the same frying pan, add another TBSP of oil if necessary, and add the spiced/herbed fish. Cook over medium-low heat about three minutes on each side or until done.

. . . .

Serving Suggestion: Serve as is or top fish with fresh guacamole. Cooking it this way reminds me of fish tacos from Baja.

. . . .

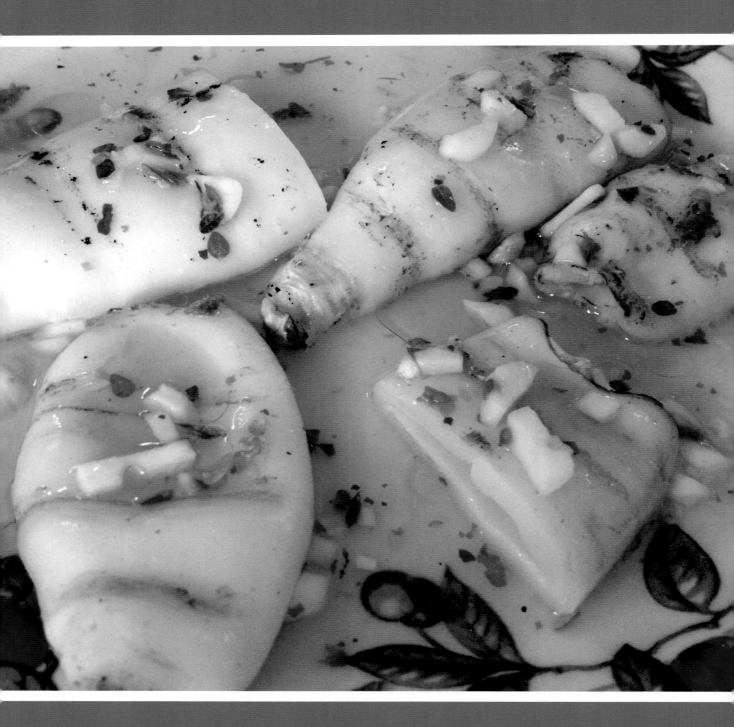

FRESH CALAMARI

(GF, SF, DF, NF, ED)

Prep time: 5 minutes

Cook time: 5 minutes

Serves 2

Ingredients

Half a pound of calamari tubes (2 inches or less), rings, and/or tentacles
(I recommend fresh calamari, but you can use frozen.)

1–2 cloves of garlic

1 teaspoon of dried oregano (fresh is okay, too)

1–2 teaspoons of red pepper flakes (or 1 small chili pepper)

2 small-medium tomatoes or half a package of cherry tomatoes, (optional)

EVOO

Salt to taste

Preparation

1. Roughly chop tomatoes. Finely chop or press garlic. Finely chop chili pepper if using.

2. Heat EVOO in a frying pan over medium heat. Add garlic and red pepper flakes, and sauté for one minute.

3. Mix in calamari and tomatoes, and sauté for two to three minutes or until done, adding salt after a minute or so.

4. Serve immediately.

Note: If you use larger calamari tubes, a longer cooking time may be necessary.

. . . .

Serving Suggestion: Serve over buckwheat pasta or as a protein source alongside one or two vegetable dishes.

. . . .

TUNA TARTARE OVER ARUGULA

(GF, SF, DF, NF)

Prep time: 30 minutes (plus one hour to marinade recommended)

Cook time: 0

Serves 4

Ingredients

- 2 pounds fresh sushi grade tuna, chopped into 1/2-inch cubes or smaller (I prefer ~1 cm. cubes.)
- 3/4 cup of EVOO
- Zest of 2 lemons* (organic!)
- Juice of 2–3 lemons (2/3 cup)
- Fresh ginger, ~2-inch piece, chopped
- Salt and pepper to taste
- 2 tablespoons poblano or jalapeño pepper
- Truffle oil for drizzling
- Hot sesame oil (optional)
- 1 tablespoon sesame seeds (optional, but recommended)
- 1/4 teaspoon wasabi powder (optional, but recommended)
- Arugula
- 2 avocados

Preparation

1. Mix first seven ingredients in a bowl. Add sesame seeds and wasabi powder if desired. I prefer to let it sit in the fridge for about one hour for flavors to settle in, but eat immediately if you're in a hurry.

2. Place desired amount of arugula onto your plate, top with chopped avocado and tuna tartare. Drizzle with truffle oil, and serve with quality gourmet potato chips or similar.

*Tip: zest lemons before slicing them.

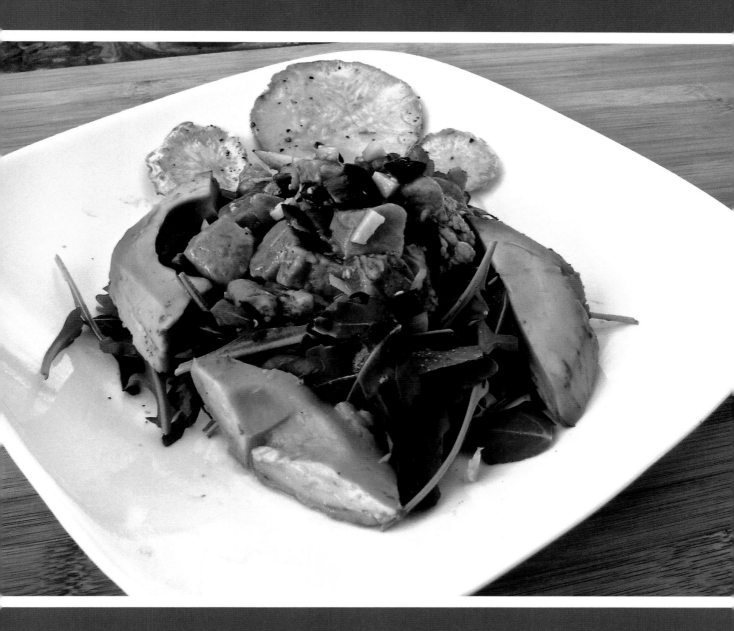

CHICKEN WINGS WITH DRY RUB

(GF, SF, DF, NF, ED)

Prep time: 10 minutes

Cook time: 25–30 minutes (depending on cooking temperature and parts used)

Serves 4

Ingredients

2 1/2 pounds chicken parts of your choice

1–2 teaspoons (start with 1 tsp. if you like it mildly flavored) of each of the following ground spices unless otherwise noted:

> Ginger
>
> Turmeric
>
> Cumin
>
> Coriander
>
> Cayenne
>
> 1/2 teaspoon black pepper
>
> 1/2 teaspoon salt
>
> 1/4 teaspoon cinnamon

Preparation

1. Preheat oven to 350°F* or preheat your grill. In a small bowl, mix ginger, cumin, coriander, turmeric, cayenne, salt, pepper, and cinnamon if using.

2. Sprinkle some of the mix on each piece of chicken and press into the chicken on both sides.

3. Place chicken in oven-proof glass or stainless steel pan, and bake for 15 minutes, and then broil on high (keeping rack in same place) for eight minutes or until crispy and done. If they are not crisp, you can turn the oven to low broil for another two to three minutes. You can also bake for 20 minutes, flipping once during cooking. (This is for wings—adjust cooking time as needed for breasts, legs, or thighs.)* Cooking time for the grill is essentially the same as for the oven, but occasional flipping is necessary.

Remove from oven, and let sit five minutes. There is no need to add oil to the pan. The chicken will make its own juices.

*Alternative cooking times and temperatures—You can also bake wings at 300°F for 30 minutes or 375°F for 15 minutes. Thighs at 350°F should bake for ~20–25 minutes and then broil on high for 5 to 8 minutes or until done.

Note: Prepare vegetable dish while meat is cooking.

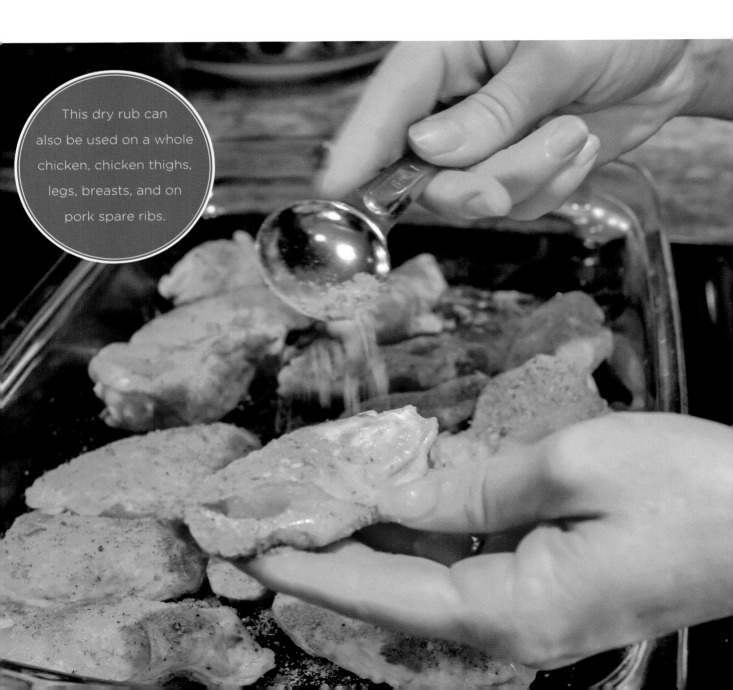

This dry rub can also be used on a whole chicken, chicken thighs, legs, breasts, and on pork spare ribs.

LEMON CHICKEN

(GF, SF, DF, NF, ED)

Prep time: 10 minutes

Cook time: 10 minutes

Serves 4

Ingredients

2 pounds chicken breasts (pounded is preferable)

Freshly squeezed lemon juice from 2-3 lemons

1 teaspoon paprika

Salt and pepper to taste

Fresh parsley to garnish (optional)

Preparation

1. Mix paprika, salt, and pepper in a small bowl. If time and desire permit, use a meat tenderizer to pound chicken breasts to 1/4-inch thickness (this will make meat more tender and allow it to cook faster but is not necessary). Sprinkle each piece with the spice mixture to taste.

2. Heat a large, heavy skillet over medium heat, and add half the amount of freshly squeezed lemon juice. Once heated, add half the chicken. For tenderized chicken, cook one minute on each side to brown, then reduce heat to medium-low and continue to cook chicken two minutes on each side or until done (cooking time depends on how thin the chicken is). Cooking time will be longer if not tenderized.

3. Repeat with remaining lemon and chicken. Garnish with fresh parsley, and serve immediately.

LAMB LOLLIPOPS

(GF, SF, DF, NF, ED)

Prep time: 10 minutes (plus 15 minutes–24 hours for marinating)

Cook time: 10–15 minutes (2x 6–8 minutes)

Serves 4

Ingredients

12–16 lamb lollipops (small chops found at the butcher, or you can buy
two racks of lamb and slice into individual chops)

3 lemons

4 large garlic cloves

Black pepper to taste

Preparation

1. Chop garlic and squeeze lemons. Marinate lamb chops for 15 minutes–24
hours in the juice of three lemons, four large garlic cloves, and black pepper.
Refrigerate if marinating longer than 15 minutes.

2. If it's been refrigerated, bring lamb almost to room temperature. Heat a
frying pan over medium or medium-low heat, and cook lamb three to four
minutes each side. Cook in two to three batches so as not to overcrowd pan.
No oil is necessary in the pan.

3. Serve immediately with your favorite side dishes.

GRASS-FED FILET MIGNON

(GF, SF, DF, NF, ED)

Prep time: 5 minutes

Cook time: 20–25 minutes

Serves 2

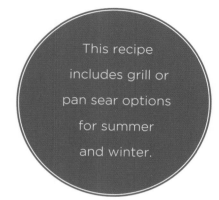

This recipe includes grill or pan sear options for summer and winter.

Ingredients

2 grass-fed filets

1 garlic clove

Salt and pepper to taste

Preparation

1. Rub with garlic clove, and sprinkle with S&P (this can be done ahead of time or just before cooking). Bring meat to almost room temperature just before cooking. Add what's left of the garlic clove to the pan while cooking.

2. Heat oven-proof skillet over medium heat until hot, and then pan sear filets for two minutes on each side.

3. Place skillet in 200°F oven for 10–20 minutes depending on how you like it cooked.

Alternate cooking method: You can also use this recipe on the grill. Cook over medium-high grill for one to two minutes each side (be careful not to burn), then lower heat and cook an additional five to ten minutes.

Tip: Prepare veggies/side dishes while meat is cooking.

Serving Suggestion: I recommend serving beef with leafy greens, such as chard, kale, and a green salad in the summer.

GRASS-FED STEAK TIPS

(GF, SF, DF, NF, ED)

Prep time: 5 minutes

Cook time: 10–15 minutes on grill; 15 minutes indoors

Serves 4

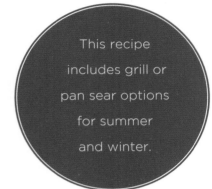

This recipe includes grill or pan sear options for summer and winter.

Ingredients

2 pounds grass-fed steak tips

1 clove of garlic

Salt and pepper to taste

Preparation for grill (BBQ)

1. Rub meat with salt, pepper, and garlic (this can be done ahead of time or just before cooking). Bring meat close to room temperature just before cooking.

2. Preheat grill with two burners on. (If using charcoal grill, rake coals to one side.)

3. Once grill is hot, turn off one burner. Place steak tips over the burner that is still on, and cook over medium-high flame for two minutes on each side (or directly over the coals) with lid closed.

4. Move meat to the part of the grill that is not lit, and cook for five to seven minutes. There is no need to flip. If the tips are thin, do not cook for more than five minutes. I also cook thick tips for only five minutes because I like them medium rare, and grass-fed beef can overcook much faster than commercially farmed beef. Plus, you can always put them back on the heat if they are undercooked.

5. Remove from grill, and let sit five minutes before cutting into them.

Preparation for stove/oven

1. Rub meat with salt, pepper, and garlic. Bring meat to room temperature.

2. Preheat oven to 200°F. Heat an oven-proof skillet over high flame. Pan sear steak tips for two minutes on each side.

3. Place skillet directly into oven, and cook about ten minutes per pound or until the internal temperature reads 125°F. Do not overcook. Let meat sit five minutes before cutting.

· ·

Serving Suggestion: Serve steak with fresh potato salad with green beans (recipe on page 119) and a green salad.

· ·

TWISTED TACOS

(GF, SF, NF)

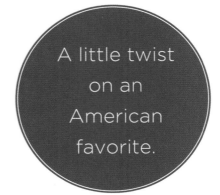

A little twist on an American favorite.

Prep time: 10 minutes

Cook time: 10–12 minutes

Serves 2–4

Ingredients

1 pound grass-fed ground beef

1-inch piece of fresh ginger

1 teaspoon coriander

8 whole cloves (slightly crushed or broken in half if desired and if time permits)

10–15 peppercorns (or ~2 tsp. ground black pepper)*

Salt to taste

Small amount of butter for sautéing (1/2 tablespoon)

1 head of large leaf lettuce

2 tomatoes

Preparation

1. Wash and dry two large lettuce leaves per person. Set aside.

2. Melt a small amount of butter in a large frying pan. Add all spices and sauté for ~one minute.

3. Add beef, and mix with spices well. Cook on medium-low for ~ten minutes or until done, stirring occasionally.

4. While the beef is cooking, chop or slice tomatoes.

5. Plate the lettuce and add desired amount of beef and tomatoes on top. Roll and eat like a taco.

* If the thought of biting into a whole peppercorn doesn't suit you, I suggest using ground black pepper instead: ~2 teaspoons or to taste.

· ·

Serving Suggestion: This dish makes a great stuffing for bell peppers (see recipe on page 85).

· ·

SESAME PORK CHOPS

(GF, SF, DF, NF, ED)

Prep time: 5–10 minutes

Cook time: 30 minutes

Serves 4

Ingredients

4 pork chops

1/4 cup sesame seeds

1–2 tablespoons of high-quality Dijon mustard

2 cloves of garlic, pressed or finely chopped

(can also use ~1 tsp. garlic paste or garlic powder)

1 tablespoon of your favorite dried herb

(oregano, thyme, herbs de Provence, or rosemary)

Salt and pepper to taste

Preparation

1. Preheat oven to 350°F.

2. On a sheet of wax paper or a large plate, mix sesame seeds, garlic, herbs, salt, and pepper into a pile.

3. Rub each pork chop with a thin layer of mustard, and dip each into the above mix.

4. Place the chops in an oven-proof pan and bake for 20 minutes.

5. Turn oven to broil (keep rack in place), and continue cooking until just brown and cooked through or for about another ten minutes, depending on thickness.

Note: Prepare vegetables/side dish while the meat is cooking.

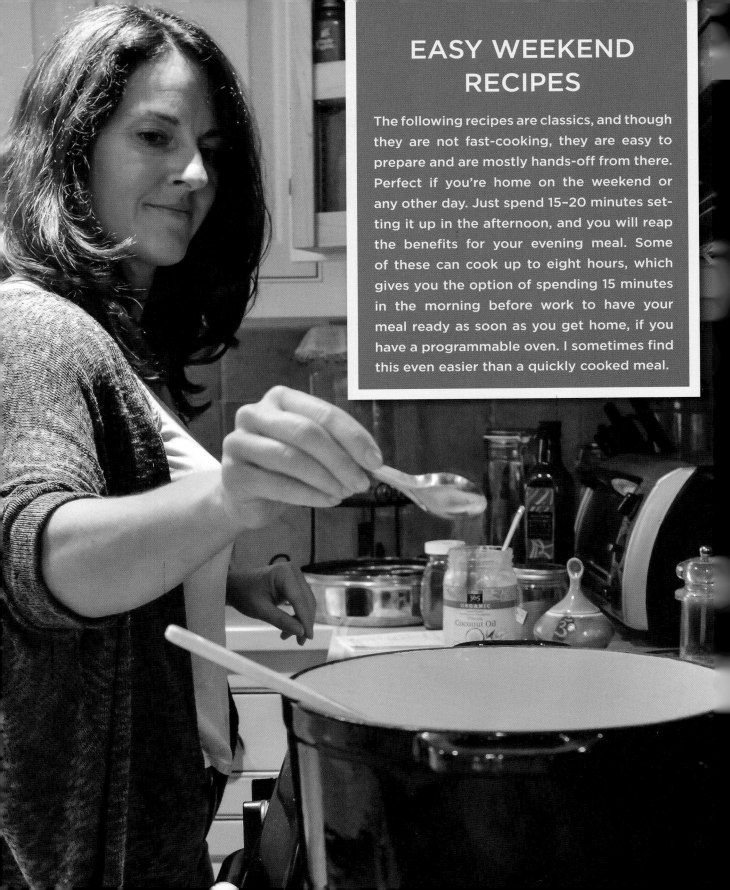

EASY WEEKEND RECIPES

The following recipes are classics, and though they are not fast-cooking, they are easy to prepare and are mostly hands-off from there. Perfect if you're home on the weekend or any other day. Just spend 15–20 minutes setting it up in the afternoon, and you will reap the benefits for your evening meal. Some of these can cook up to eight hours, which gives you the option of spending 15 minutes in the morning before work to have your meal ready as soon as you get home, if you have a programmable oven. I sometimes find this even easier than a quickly cooked meal.

HERBED TURKEY THIGHS

(GF, SF, DF, NF, ED)

This recipe is adapted from The Whole-Food Guide to Overcoming Irritable Bowel Syndrome *by Laura J. Knoff, NC.*

Prep time: 15 minutes

Cook time: 1, 1-1/2, 3, 5, or 8 hours, depending on temperature

Serves 4

Ingredients

2–3 turkey thighs (I use skinless, approximately 3 pounds total.)

1 bunch of carrots (about 6 medium or large carrots)

Dulse granules (see resources)

2 cloves of garlic

Generous amount of fresh or dried herbs, such as sage, oregano, parsley, or thyme (I use 8–10 freshly picked sage leaves from my garden, and they are delicious!)

1 small onion (optional)

0–8 oz. broth or water (optional and dependent on cooking time)

Preparation

1. Preheat oven to desired temperature (see step five to determine temp).

2. Scrub or peel carrots, and peel onion. Chop onion and carrots into medium chunks. Chop herbs if using fresh. Place carrots on the bottom of a glass or stainless steel baking dish.

3. Place the turkey thighs skin-side up on top of the carrots and sprinkle with dulse. Press garlic on top, and cover with herbs and onion.

4. If cooking for five hours or more, add enough broth or water to cover bottom of pan to about a 1/2 inch deep (~8 oz.). If cooking three hours or less, the addition of liquid is not necessary, but I usually add it anyway because I love broth.

5. If cooking for one hour, set oven to 350°F; for one and a half hours, set oven to 300°; for three hours, set oven to 275°F; for five hours, set oven to 250°F. If cooking longer than five hours, set oven to 200°F–225°F. Eight hours at 200°F works well and is convenient to set up overnight or while you're at work (if you have an automatic oven shut-off).

6. Cover the baking dish securely with aluminum foil and place in the oven, or use a slow cooker on medium or low. When done, the meat should be so juicy it falls apart.

SLOW-COOKED BABY BACK RIBS

(GF, SF, DF, NF)

Prep time: 5–10 minutes

Cook time: 4 hours

Serves 4

Ingredients

1 large rack of baby back ribs

1 tablespoon ground espresso (freshly ground is best)

1–2 teaspoons cayenne

2 teaspoons paprika

1 teaspoon salt

2–3 cloves of garlic (optional, can substitute with garlic powder)

Preparation

1. Preheat oven to 225°F.

2. Mix all ingredients except ribs in a small bowl. Rub the mix onto the ribs.

3. Place ribs in stainless steel pan, meaty-side down. Cover with foil, and cook four hours.

4. Remove from oven, and let sit for 15 minutes before serving.

BEEF STEW

(GF, SF, DF, NF)

Prep time: 20 minutes

Cook time: 2 hours

Ingredients

- 2 1/2 pounds beef sirloin, cubed into approximately 1-inch pieces *
- 6 medium carrots
- 2–3 Yukon potatoes (or 10 fingerling potatoes)
- 8 ounces of baby bella or crimini mushrooms
- 1 bell pepper (I like to use red or orange.)
- 2–3 cloves of garlic
- Green beans (can use fresh or frozen 8 oz.), optional
- 1 cup of red wine (The flavor will come out so use a decent wine.)
- 1 TBSP high-quality mustard or horseradish (optional)
- 1 cup organic beef or mushroom broth or 1/4–1/2 cup water (if necessary)
- 1 bay leaf
- Dried or fresh herbs, such as thyme, rosemary, oregano, parsley, or herbs de Provence
- Salt and pepper

* You can use "stew meat," but it is not as juicy as sirloin. I buy sirloin steak tips and chop them myself (you can also have the butcher chop them for you). No matter what cut of beef you choose, please make sure it's grass-fed!

Preparation

1. Chop mushrooms and garlic; set aside. Chop meat if necessary.**

2. Sprinkle a small amount of S&P on chopped meat. Heat a large stew pot on medium-high, and sear meat in two or more batches so as only to layer the bottom of pan and not have the meat piled on top of each other. Brown the meat on each side, and then promptly remove and brown the next batch. Remove last batch from the pot.

3. Add garlic and mushrooms to the pot, and sauté until the mushrooms are soft and liquid is present. Add meat back in, plus wine, broth, bay leaf, herbs, and mustard or horseradish and simmer, covered, on very low for 50 minutes to an hour (one hour for non-grass-fed beef).

4. While the meat is cooking, chop carrots and potatoes into 3/4–1-inch cubes and set aside.

5. After the meat has cooked for 50–60 minutes, add carrots, potatoes, and green beans. Continue to simmer another 30 minutes.

6. Add bell pepper and continue to simmer another 30 minutes or until everything is tender.

**You can choose to chop all the veggies in the beginning if you prefer to walk away from the kitchen while the meat is cooking. Chopping the carrots and potatoes while the meat is cooking saves about 10–15 minutes of overall time.

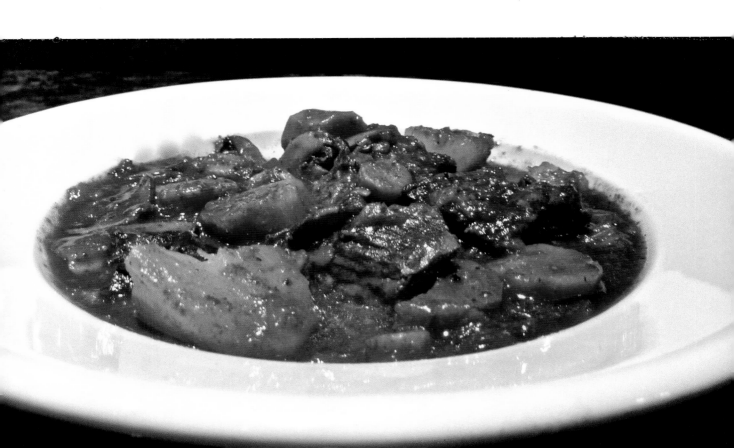

TRADITIONAL, AND SO SIMPLE, POT ROAST

(GF, SF, DF, NF, ED)

Prep time: 15 minutes

Cook time: 2 1/2 –3 hours

Serves 4

Ingredients

3–4 pound pot roast

2–3 cloves of garlic, chopped or not

Herbs (such as herbs de Provence, oregano, rosemary, and thyme)

1 bay leaf

Salt and pepper to taste

Red wine and/or beef or mushroom broth, ~2 cups total

Purified water (if necessary)

4–6 medium carrots

8-ounce package of mushrooms

Preparation

1. Preheat oven to 250°F.

2. Roughly chop carrots and mushrooms, and set aside.

3. Brown the roast on all sides over medium-high heat in a Dutch oven or ceramic pot that can transfer to the oven. Browning all sides takes about three minutes total.

4. Add garlic, herbs, bay leaf, salt, pepper, and enough liquid to cover the roast halfway. You can use a combination of red wine, beef or mushroom broth, and water.

5. Add carrots and mushrooms.

6. Cover the pot and place in the oven. Remove after two and a half to three hours, and let sit for 10–15 minutes before serving.

Note: You can also use this recipe to cook beef short ribs. They are delicious when slow cooked at 250–275°F for four to five hours.

ROASTED CHICKEN AND ROOT VEGETABLES

(GF, SF, DF, NF, ED)

Prep time: 15 minutes

Cook time: 1–2 hours (your choice)

Serves 4

Ingredients

    1 whole chicken

    1 bunch of your favorite root veggie or a mixture

      (carrots, turnips, parsnips, rutabaga, and potatoes)

    1 lemon

    2 tablespoons herbs de Provence

      (or a mix of thyme, oregano, rosemary, lavender, and marjoram)

    1–2 cloves of garlic, chopped

    1 bay leaf

    Salt and pepper to taste

    4 ounces of water if necessary

Preparation

1. Preheat oven to 325°F if cooking for two hours (recommended if time permits) or 400°F if cooking for one hour (suggested only if time does not allow for two-hour cooking time).

2. Wash root vegetables and peel if necessary (if carrots are from a trusted source, organic, and scrubbed well, you may not need to peel them). Slice veggies and place around perimeter of roasting pan along with any desired organ meat from within the cavity of the chicken (be sure to remove and use or discard organ meat from within the chicken).

3. Place chicken in center of veggie-lined roasting pan and dress each side of the chicken liberally with lemon juice, garlic, herbs, and S&P. Also sprinkle herbs and lemon juice on veggies. Place bay leaf, remaining lemon juice, spent lemon rind, and S&P in the cavity of the chicken.

4. Cook chicken breast-side up for one to two hours depending on temperature chosen. Don't overcook. If cooking for one hour, check chicken after 30 minutes and baste with juices if desired, or add a few ounces of water to bottom of pan if it's looking dry. Juices will usually form naturally

from the chicken and lemon, so you can also check again after 45 minutes and decide whether or not to add water then. I usually don't find it necessary to add water.

5. Once chicken is cooked, remove from oven and let sit for 15 minutes before cutting.

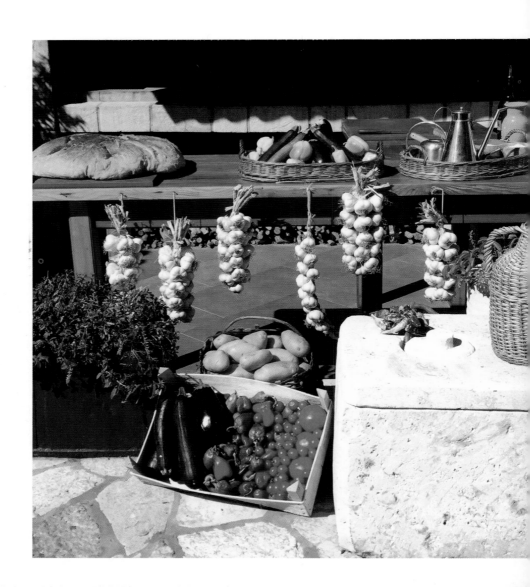

VEGETABLE

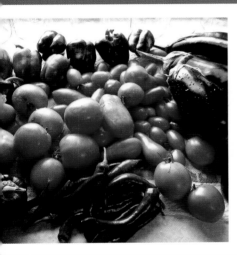 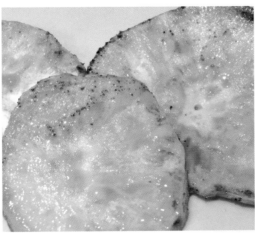 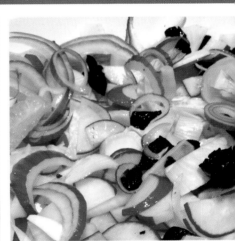

SIDE DISHES

There are so many delicious, nutritious vegetables available, and I recommend trying all of them at some point. In the meantime, here are some staples that are tasty and easy to make.

For evenings that you're really in a hurry, I recommend simply steaming some fresh vegetables, then drizzling with olive oil, salt, and pepper (see the *Asparagus, Simply Cooked* recipe on page 93). Having a few choices of high-quality, organic, frozen vegetables such as peas and green beans is helpful in a pinch, too, but steaming fresh veggies is quite fast and easy. Some quick options are asparagus, broccoli, green beans, and peas. Washing and chopping takes about five minutes, and steaming takes five to ten minutes. For broccoli, I sometimes add washed, chopped florets to boiling water, then gently boil for three minutes, and drain immediately. It can be that simple. Toss with EVOO and salt and pepper, and you'll be nourishing your family in no time.

In the summertime, when we tend to eat more raw vegetables, keeping a box or two of prewashed salad greens makes for a quickly prepared salad. Toss in some cherry tomatoes (no chopping required) and whatever else you like, and voilà. Olivia's is my favorite brand of salad greens. They tend to be the freshest and cleanest.

Serving size applies to the vegetable as a side dish unless otherwise stated.

ODE TO MY ITALIAN HERITAGE: STUFFED ARTICHOKES

(GF, SF, VG)

Prep time: 15 minutes

Cook time: 20–45 minutes

Serves 4

Ingredients

    4 large artichokes

    2 large cloves of garlic, pressed or finely chopped

    2 cups of hazelnut meal or almond meal

    Juice of half a lemon

    Sprinkle of Italian herbs, such as oregano and parsley (dried works best here)

    Grated Parmigiano-Reggiano (Parmesan) cheese (optional)

    EVOO

    Salt and pepper to taste

Preparation

1. Rinse artichokes, and cut off the stems and the tops about 1 1/2 inches down. You can keep the stems and throw them in the pot—sometimes they are tender enough to eat, and sometimes they are too stringy, in which case I throw them away. You won't know until after cooking. Once the tops are trimmed, spread the leaves and rinse the artichokes again, getting in between the leaves as much as possible. Shake out the excess water.

2. In a bowl, combine the nut meal, garlic, herbs, cheese, lemon, and S&P. Mix well and add EVOO as needed until it is well formed in a way where you can easily stuff the artichokes without crumbs flying everywhere. As you add the EVOO, mix with your hands by squishing (kneading) the meal instead of stirring with a utensil. This will create the best texture without requiring too much oil.

3. Using a small spoon and/or your hands, place stuffing within some of the leaves of each artichoke and top each with additional stuffing.

4. Fill a large pot with two inches of water, and carefully place artichokes in the pot. Cover pot, bring to a boil, then reduce heat and simmer for 35–45 minutes or until you can easily pull a leaf from the artichoke. For faster cooking, you can use a pressure cooker—prepare the pot and artichokes the

same way, but cook ~15 minutes once the pot whistles (it usually takes two to five minutes for the pot to whistle). If there is room in the pot, go ahead and toss in the stems if desired. When the artichokes are done, check the tenderness of the stems and decide if you want to eat them with a squeeze of lemon.

To eat artichokes: Pull leaves and scrape the meat off the tip with teeth (according to my great-uncle, and I agree, this works best if you hold the leaf upside down). Once you get to the *choke,* scrape off the *whiskers* with a spoon or fork and eat the heart, which is the most delicious part.

Stuffed artichokes are traditionally made with bread crumbs, but I've found nut meals to be a tasty and healthy substitute.

• •

When I was a little girl, my grandmother and my great-uncle taught me how to eat an artichoke: turn the leaf upside down and scrape the meat off with your teeth. We had many laughs while we enjoyed these delicious, nutritious vegetables. For the health benefits, taste, and, of course, the fun, these are my favorite!

• •

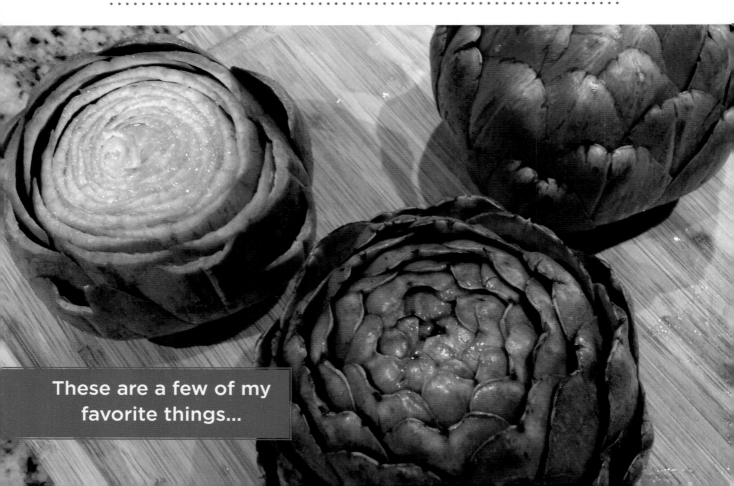

These are a few of my favorite things...

STUFFED PEPPERS

(GF, SF, DF, VG)

Prep time: 5 minutes initial prep time; 10 minutes while peppers cook

Cook time: 40 minutes

Serves: 4 as a side dish or 2 as a meal

A pepper can be stuffed with many different things. Here is one of my favorite stuffing recipes, plus a few suggestions about how to use leftovers to stuff peppers.

Ingredients

2 red bell peppers (or any pepper large enough to stuff)

2 cups of almond or hazelnut meal
(1/2 cup per half pepper, depending on size of pepper)

2–3 cloves of garlic, crushed or finely chopped

1/2 cup of chopped fresh parsley (or 1 tablespoon dried)

EVOO to desired consistency

Salt and pepper to taste

Preparation

1. Preheat oven to 375°F.

2. Slice the peppers in half lengthwise and cut out the fleshy parts and seeds.

3. Place peppers in oven-proof baking dish, drizzle with a small amount of EVOO, and bake for 30 minutes.

4. Meanwhile, prepare the nut meal stuffing by adding nut meal, garlic, parsley, and S&P to a bowl and mix. Then gradually stir in EVOO until the mixture is moist and not crumbly. Mixing with your hands will help the nut meal absorb the EVOO so you can use less.

5. After the peppers have cooked for 30 minutes, add the stuffing and continue to cook until the peppers are soft and the stuffing is warm for about another ten minutes.

6. Drizzle with EVOO if desired and serve.

Alternative stuffing suggestions: If you have leftover spiced quinoa (page 122), quinoa with greens (page 116), twisted taco meat (page 71), or saffron rice (page 117), you can use these to stuff your pepper.

Take the leftovers out of the refrigerator just before you begin the preparation above. Follow steps one through three above, then add the filling (which should be almost room temperature) and continue to bake as instructed in steps five and six above. You can also make any of these fresh while the pepper is cooking in step three, and stuff the pepper as instructed above in step five. In this case, I recommend omitting the pepper in the spiced quinoa recipe.

OKRA

(GF, SF, DF, NF, VG, ED)

Prep time: 10-15 minutes

Cook time: 15 minutes

Serves 4

Ingredients

- 1 pound fresh okra (frozen will work, too)
- 1 tablespoon EVOO
- 1 teaspoon mustard seeds
- 1 teaspoon cumin seeds
- 1/2 teaspoon salt
- 1/2 green chili (optional)

Preparation

1. Trim ends of okra and chop into 1/4-1/2-inch pieces. Chop green chili and remove seeds if desired.

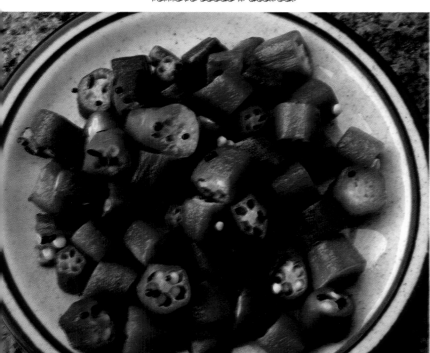

2. Heat EVOO in a pan over medium-low to medium heat. Add cumin seeds and mustard seeds. Sauté until you hear the seeds gently pop. Add salt and chili, and sauté for one to two minutes.

3. Add okra, cover and simmer for 15 minutes or until tender. Stir occasionally during cooking.

Tip: If you can't find okra stocked in your local grocery store, try Whole Foods or an Indian grocery store.

ZUCCHINI, INDIAN STYLE

(GF, SF, DF, NF, VG, ED)

Prep time: 10 minutes

Cook time: 10–15 minutes

Serves 4

Ingredients

2 medium–large zucchini

1/2 teaspoon each of cumin and coriander powder
(or 1 teaspoon of *dhana jiru**)

1/2–1 teaspoon turmeric powder

1 large clove of garlic

Pinch of salt

2 tablespoons of EVOO. More if necessary during cooking.

Preparation

1. Cut zucchini into 1/4-inch slices, and then chop slices in half (make a stack of slices and cut through the middle to cut them in half quickly).

2. Heat EVOO in a sauté or frying pan over low-medium heat. Add cumin and coriander (or *dhana jiru**) and turmeric, and sauté for about one minute.

3. While the spices are sautéing and tantalizing you with their aroma, finely chop the garlic and add it to the pan. You can also use a garlic press and press directly into the pan.

4. Add zucchini and a pinch of salt, and stir well. Keep the heat on low and cook until the zucchini becomes slightly translucent and soft, but not mushy, for about eight minutes. Stir occasionally during cooking, and add EVOO a teaspoon at a time if the zucchini sticks to the pan.

* *Dhana jiru* is a combination of cumin and coriander widely used in Indian cooking.

BALANCED EGGPLANT

(GF, SF, DF, NF, VG)

Prep time: 10 minutes

Cook time: 15 minutes

Serves 4

Ingredients

- 2 medium eggplants
- 1 teaspoon cumin seeds (powder okay if you don't have seeds)
- 1 teaspoon mustard seeds
- 1 teaspoon coriander powder
- 1/2 teaspoon turmeric powder (or ~1-inch piece of fresh turmeric, chopped)
- 1/2 teaspoon salt
- 4 tablespoons EVOO

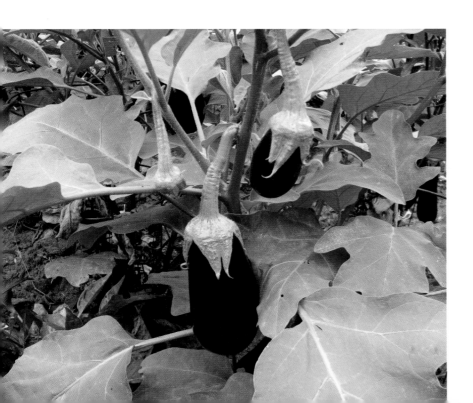

Preparation

1. Peel eggplant and chop into 3/4-inch cubes.

2. Add 2 TBSP EVOO to a large frying pan over low-medium heat. Add cumin seeds, mustard seeds, and turmeric. Stirring occasionally, sauté until you hear the seeds pop (about two minutes). Stir in coriander and salt, and then add eggplant.

3. Immediately after mixing in the eggplant, add another TBSP of EVOO and gently mix.

4. Turn heat to low, cover, and simmer for 12–15 minutes or until soft. Stir occasionally, about every five minutes, during cooking and add remaining TBSP of EVOO if necessary.

· ·

Eggplant has been one of my greatest teachers. Indeed, anything can be a teacher if we are paying attention. Eggplant is one of my favorite vegetables, and as a young adult I ate it ad nauseam. Eggplant Parmesan was a favorite to make at home and to eat out. It was a dish surrounded in romance and a reason for my husband to feel that "this woman's a keeper." In our early years we would take long lunches and get to know each other over a dish of eggplant siciliano at a local Italian eatery. A visit to Randazzo's in Miami for the eggplant parm became a tradition while visiting my daughter in college. But as time went on, eggplant liked me less and less. Or maybe it liked me so much that it enjoyed hanging out in my body like a lead balloon. Then one day—I believe it was day three of eating eggplant in some form or another—I took a bite and my throat felt scratchy. Red flag. Now I'm listening. I stopped eating eggplant completely for about a year. During that year I learned about food rotation, balancing foods from the perspective of Ayurveda, and most importantly, I learned that just because I eliminated gluten, that didn't mean I could eat everything else. Anyone can be sensitive to anything, and your inner detective must always be vigilant. This is especially true once you clean up your diet because you will likely feel what's going on with your body more than you did before. I was eating too much eggplant and in combination with the wrong foods (tomato sauce, garlic, and cheese). During my eggplant hiatus, I took an Ayurveda cooking class and, wouldn't you know, eggplant was on the menu. I learned what spices balance the hot nature of eggplant to make it more digestible. The result was delicious, and I felt great after eating it. I still only eat eggplant sparingly, but when I do, I balance it out with the cooling nature of coriander, and it's true love again.

· ·

SAUTÉED GREENS

(GF, SF, DF, NF, VG, ED)

> Sautéed greens taste great and are a quick and easy way to get nutrients into your body.

Prep time: 10 minutes

Cook time: 10 minutes

Serves 4

Ingredients

1 bunch of selected green (Swiss chard, kale, mustard greens, collard greens, spinach, broccoli rabe—rapini—or any similar green work well for this recipe)

2 tablespoons of EVOO

1–2 cloves of garlic (optional)*

Salt and pepper to taste

Preparation

1. Wash and spin greens, and then chop into large bite-size pieces. Chop garlic if using.

2. Gently heat EVOO in a large frying pan or wide pot. If using garlic, sauté for about one minute, and then add S&P to taste (start with 1/2 tsp. if you're unsure).

3. Add greens, in batches if necessary, and sauté until just tender but still bright green, for about two to four minutes (chard and spinach will cook very quickly). Turn greens frequently while cooking so the ones on the bottom don't overcook and wilt.

*I use garlic for the less flavorful greens like chard and leave it out with spicier greens like mustard greens or broccoli rabe.

BRUSSELS SPROUTS

(GF, SF, DF*, VG)

Prep time: 10 minutes

Cook time: 15 minutes

Serves 4

Ingredients

> 1 pound Brussels sprouts
>
> 3 tablespoons pine nuts
>
> 2 cloves of garlic
>
> 2–3 tablespoons of unsalted butter (You can use EVOO if you prefer.)*
>
> Salt and pepper to taste

Preparation

1. Pull outer leaves off sprouts if they are loose, and chop stems off. Wash and slice sprouts in half lengthwise. Chop or press garlic.

2. Heat butter or EVOO over medium-low in a large skillet, and then add remaining ingredients. Try to place sprouts inside pan in an even layer. If this is not possible (for me it's usually not), just stir occasionally so they cook evenly. If the sprouts are in one layer, you do not need to stir, but check once during cooking to be sure they are not sticking. Add more butter or EVOO if necessary.

3. Cook until just tender and barely turning golden brown (about 15 minutes).

Alternate cooking method: Preheat oven to 350°F. Add sliced sprouts, garlic, pine nuts, and salt and pepper to a large bowl and toss evenly with EVOO or melted butter. Pour into a baking dish, arrange sprouts in one layer, and bake for 15–20 minutes or until just tender and golden brown.

* This dish is dairy-free if you use EVOO instead of butter.

ASPARAGUS, SIMPLY COOKED

(GF, SF, DF, NF, VG, ED)

Prep time: 5 minutes

Cook time: 10 minutes

Serves 2

> I've included this recipe to remind you that eating real food is simple, and you don't need to make an exotic or new recipe every day. On the busiest of days, this is what I turn to since it is easy to prepare, delicious, and fresh.

Ingredients

1 bunch of asparagus*

Juice of half a lemon

EVOO

Salt and pepper to taste

Preparation for steamed asparagus

1. Wash asparagus and break or chop off woody ends.

2. Put in steamer, bring to boil, and then simmer about five to ten minutes until just soft but *al dente*.

3. Remove to serving dish and drizzle with EVOO, lemon, and S&P.

Preparation for grilled or roasted asparagus

1. Place asparagus in foil or grill-safe tray for grilling and cookie sheet or glass tray for roasting. Drizzle with small amount of EVOO and S&P.

2. Grill over medium heat or roast at 375°F for 10–12 minutes.

3. Remove to serving dish, and drizzle with lemon and more EVOO if desired.

*This steamed recipe also works well for broccoli or fresh peas. The grilled recipe works well for eggplant or zucchini, sliced lengthwise. Another way to cook broccoli is to add chopped broccoli to gently boiling water and cook, uncovered, for about three minutes. You want the color to remain bright green while the florets are just tender. Gently boiling broccoli is said to make it more suitable for people with thyroid disorders who are avoiding raw cruciferous vegetables.

GREEN BEANS WITH MUSTARD DRESSING

(GF, SF, DF, NF, VG, ED)

Prep time: 10 minutes

Cook time: 5–10 minutes

Serves 4

Ingredients

  1 pound fresh green beans (You can also use frozen green beans.)

  1 tablespoon Dijon mustard (more or less to taste)

  1 tablespoon EVOO

  2 sprigs of fresh thyme (or 1/2 teaspoon of dried thyme)

Preparation

1. Wash the beans, and trim the ends off. Slice beans in half.

2. Steam the beans for approximately eight minutes or until tender with a slight crunch.

3. While beans are steaming, remove leaves from stem if using fresh thyme. Whisk together the thyme, mustard, and EVOO in a small bowl and set aside.

4. When beans are cooked, transfer them to a serving dish or bowl and toss with the mustard dressing and serve.

RADICCHIO WITH FENNEL

(GF, SF, DF, NF, VG, ED)

Prep time: 5 minutes

Cook time: 8–10 minutes

Serves 2–4

Ingredients

1 bunch of radicchio

1 tablespoon fennel seeds

1 teaspoon salt

2 tablespoon EVOO

The sweet taste of fennel seeds balances out the bitter taste of radicchio in this dish.

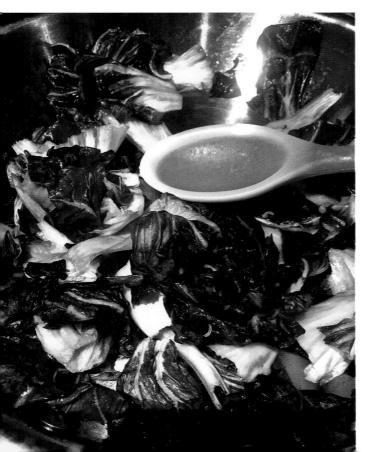

Preparation

1. Chop radicchio into ~2-inch pieces.

2. Add EVOO to large frying pan over low heat.

3. Add fennel seeds and stir for one minute.

4. Add radicchio and salt and cook until tender, about five to ten minutes. Stir occasionally.

Note: This recipe can also be used for beet greens or a combination of beet greens and radicchio. The fennel seeds add sweetness to the bitter taste of these greens.

BEETS IN BALSAMIC DRESSING

(GF, SF, DF, NF, VG, ED)

Prep time: 2 minutes before cooking; 5 minutes after cooking

Cook time: 30 minutes

Serves 4

Ingredients

1 large bunch of beets, any variety or a mix (or 2 small bunches)

1–2 tablespoon balsamic vinegar
 (works best with a thick, sweet balsamic like Rubio brand)

2 tablespoon EVOO

Sprinkling of herbs, such as oregano, thyme, or herbs de Provence

Salt and pepper to taste

Preparation

1. Get a large pot of water boiling. Remove greens (which can be saved and eaten in a salad if they are fresh), scrub beets (thoroughly if you plan to eat skin), and place in boiling water.

2. Cook at a low boil for 30 minutes or until just tender. (Cooking time depends on size of beets. They are done when you can just begin to stick them with a fork.)

3. Drain water and let beets cool enough so that you can peel them if desired. Organic, washed beets don't need to be peeled, and their skin provides added nutrients such as fiber, plus a slightly more earthy taste (beets provide fiber without skins, too). Try one unpeeled and see if you like it. You will save time if you don't have to peel the skin.

4. Cut beets in half or quarters, sprinkle with herbs, and drizzle with balsamic vinegar and EVOO. Add S&P to taste.

Alternate preparation: Preheat oven to 375°F. Peel and chop beets. Place in a roasting pan and drizzle with EVOO and herbs. Cover pan with foil and bake for 20 minutes. Place beets in a serving bowl or plate and drizzle with balsamic vinegar. Add salt and pepper to taste.

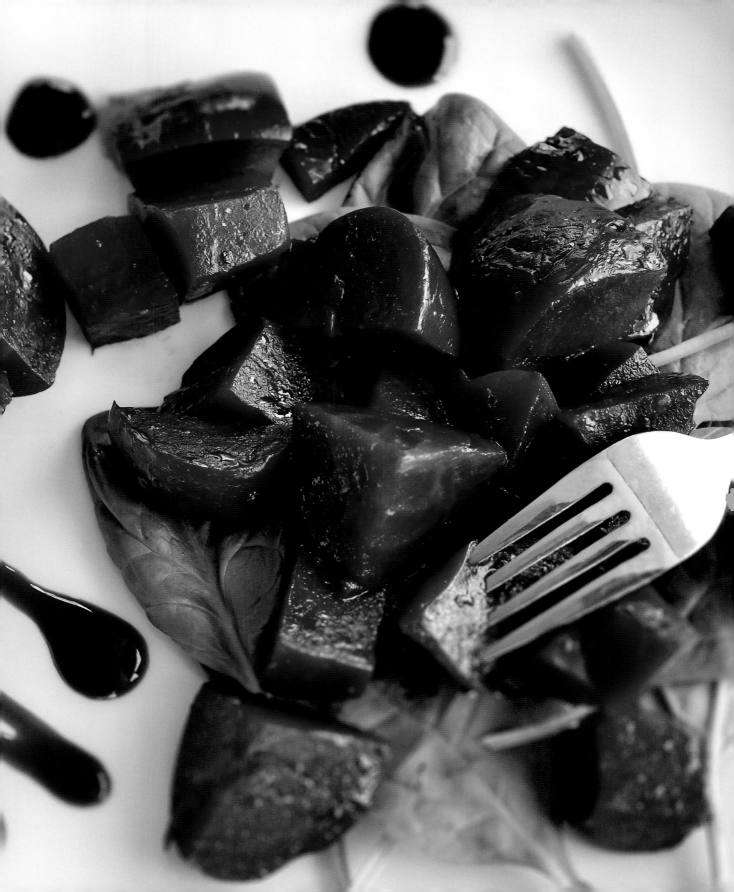

SAUTÉED PEPPERS (ODE TO RITA AND IVO)

(GF, SF, DF*, NF, VG)

Prep time: 10 minutes

Cook time: 15 minutes

Serves 4

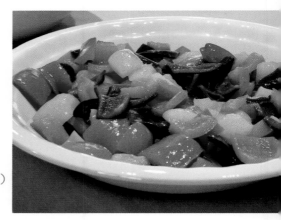

Ingredients

3 red, orange, and/or yellow bell peppers

(sometimes I throw in a poblano, too)

2 tablespoons butter

(or EVOO if you prefer or require dairy-free)

Preparation

1. Wash and slice the peppers, removing seeds. I like them chopped into 1–2-inch pieces rather than long strips, but chop to your liking.

2. Put large frying pan on low heat and add butter or EVOO. I prefer the taste with butter but use EVOO or a combo if you prefer. Once the butter is melted, add peppers. Cover and cook over low-medium heat, stirring occasionally, for 15 minutes or until tender and just beginning to caramelize.

Tip: Peppers can be served as is or over quinoa or similar grain.

· ·

In the autumn of 2006, I stayed with my friend Mary's sister Rita and her husband Ivo in Pinzolo, Italy. Everything in Italy tastes better, especially if it's home-cooked. My first evening in their home, they prepared risotto and sautéed red peppers. I'd eaten peppers 101 ways but never as simply and sweet as this. I was pleasantly surprised at how easy and delicious the sautéed peppers were and couldn't believe I'd never thought to make them this way. More often than we think, the best flavors come from the simplest preparation.

· ·

CELERY ROOT CHIPS

(GF, SF, DF, NF, VG, ED)

Prep time: 10 minutes

Cook time: 15–20 minutes

Serves 4

Ingredients

1 large celery root

Salt and pepper to taste

Paprika to taste (optional)

EVOO

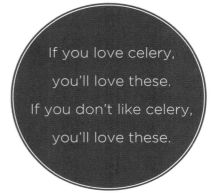

If you love celery, you'll love these. If you don't like celery, you'll love these.

Preparation

1. Preheat oven to 375°F.

2. Peel and slice the celery root into pieces just under 1/4-inch thick.

3. Arrange in a single layer in a baking dish and drizzle with EVOO, sprinkle with salt, pepper, and paprika.

4. Bake eight minutes, then flip over and bake another eight minutes or until just crisp. Or after the first eight minutes, broil on low or 375°F for the remaining eight minutes. Note: Cooking time may vary slightly from oven to oven and depending on thickness of slices.

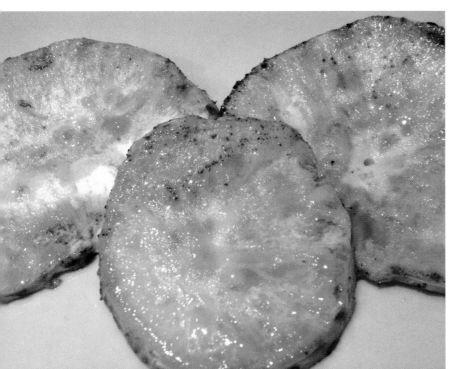

PORTABELLA MUSHROOMS

(GF, SF, NF, VG*)

Prep time: 5–10 minutes (during and after cooking)

Cook time: 5–8 minutes

Serves 4

Ingredients

    4 large portabella mushrooms (stems removed for better plating)

    1/4 cup EVOO

    1 teaspoon anchovy paste (optional)*

    2 tablespoon balsamic vinegar

    1/2 teaspoon dried thyme

    3 cups arugula

    Salt and pepper to taste

    Parmigiano-Reggiano (Parmesan) for shaving

Preparation

1. Preheat grill or preheat oven to 400°F.

2. Cook portabellas, flipping two to three times during cooking on grill or once if in oven (or bake five minutes, and then broil on low for five minutes).

3. While the portabellas are cooking, in a small bowl mix the EVOO, anchovy paste, vinegar, and thyme.

4. Once the portabellas are soft, remove them from heat, place gill-side up, and drizzle with the above dressing, leaving ~2 TBSP behind for the arugula.

5. At this point, you can leave the mushrooms to marinate for up to 30 minutes if time permits or continue on if not.

6. Toss the arugula with the remaining dressing and season with S&P.

7. Plate the arugula and top with a mushroom. Shave Parmigiano-Reggiano on top if desired.

Tip: For faster prep, just toss the arugula on each plate, top with cooked, undressed portabella and drizzle dressing on top.

SUZANNE'S PEPPERY FLORAL SALAD

(GF, SF, DF, NF, VG, ED)

Prep time: 15 minutes

Cook time: 0

Serves 2

From late spring to early autumn I make this salad from whatever is in my garden. In this case I had arugula and nasturtium ready for harvesting. These plants are easy to grow and harvest, and nasturtium makes an impressive and tasty addition to any salad.

Ingredients

Fill a salad bowl with your favorite fresh salad greens (I use arugula and nasturtium leaves)

4 large radishes, chopped

4 nasturtium flowers (can also use borage, calendula, or marigold)

Juice of 1/2 a lemon

1/4 cup of EVOO

Salt and pepper to taste

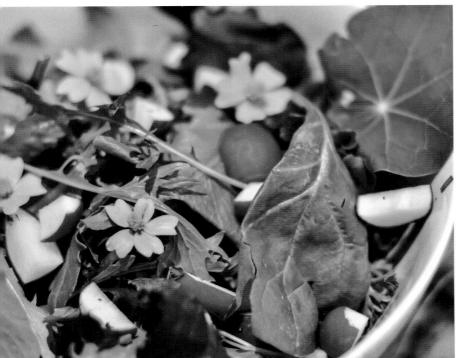

Preparation

Add all ingredients to a salad bowl in the order listed above. Enjoy!

Tip: Of the flowers listed, I find that borage has the mildest flavor and marigold has the strongest. Calendula and marigold have a somewhat bitter flavor, and nasturtium leaves and flowers have a peppery flavor.

COLORFUL SPRING SALAD

(GF, SF, DF, NF, VG, ED)

Prep time: 5 minutes

Cook time: 0

Serves 2

Ingredients

    1/2 box of Olivia's spring mix (or your favorite leafy greens)

    1/2 small head of red cabbage

    1/2 box arugula

    EVOO

    Fresh lemon juice (fresh orange can also be used)

    Salt and pepper to taste

    Avocado (optional)

    Sunflower seeds (optional)

    Edible flowers (optional)

Preparation

1. Chop the cabbage to desired size and slice the avocado if using.

2. Mix greens, cabbage, and arugula in a bowl. Add avocado and seeds if using. Top with EVOO, lemon, salt, and pepper. It tastes as good as it looks.

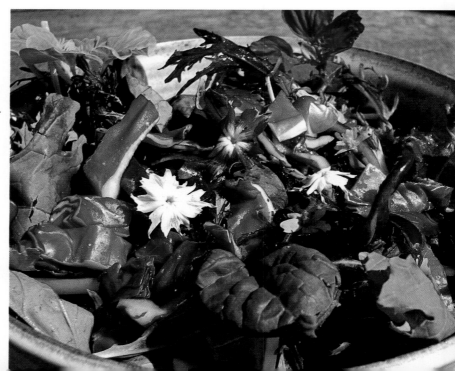

SICILIAN FENNEL AND ORANGE SALAD

(GF, SF, DF, NF, VG, ED)

Prep time: 10 minutes

Cook time: 0 minutes

Serves 4

Ingredients

> 2 navel oranges
>
> 1 large fennel bulb
>
> 1 red onion
>
> 1/2 cup radishes
>
> 1/2 cup oil cured black olives (preferably pitted)
>
> 1/4 cup EVOO (or more if desired)

Preparation

1. Remove stems from fennel and slice thinly as you would an onion.

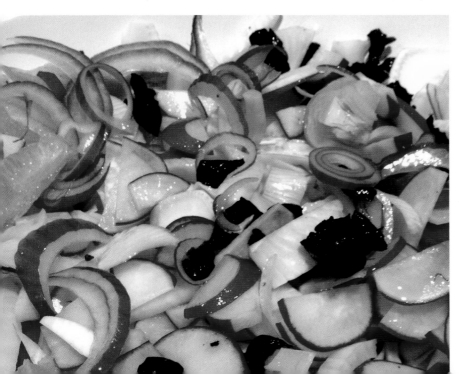

2. Slice radishes and add to fennel.

3. Thinly slice onion and add to salad.

4. Peel the orange and remove as much skin/pulp as you can. Divide and add to salad.

5. Pit olives if necessary, chop if desired (not necessary), and add to salad.

6. Pour EVOO on top and toss gently.

GREENS WRAPPED IN COCONUT

(GF, SF, DF, VG, ED*)

Prep time: 20 minutes

Cook time: 0

Makes 4 wraps

Ingredients for salad

> 1 cup chopped kale (~3 ounces)
>
> 1 cup chopped lettuce or other salad greens (~3 ounces)
>
> 1 large cucumber
>
> 1 carrot
>
> 1/2 red onion (optional)
>
> 1/4 cup sunflower seeds (optional)
>
> Black pepper to taste
>
> 4 Paleo coconut wraps (see resources)

Ingredients for dressing

> 1 avocado
>
> 2 cups fresh parsley
>
> Juice from 1 large lemon
>
> 2 cloves of garlic
>
> 5 tablespoons water
>
> 1 teaspoon salt

Preparation

1. Add all dressing ingredients except water to a Nutribullet, Vitamix, chopper, or blender. A smaller vessel, such as the Nutribullet or chopper, works best because of the small volume, but any of these will do. If you are using a blender or Vitamix, I recommend chopping the garlic first to ensure it doesn't remain as one large piece in someone's wrap.

*If you can eat coconut safely, this recipe is suitable for an elimination diet.

2. Once the ingredients are mostly blended, add 3 TBSP of water and blend. If a thinner consistency is desired, add remaining water, 1 TBSP at a time. Set dressing aside.

3. Chop the kale, lettuce, cucumber, and onion. Grate, peel, or thinly slice the carrot. I prefer to use the peeler to make thin slices as long or short as I like.

4. Add all chopped salad ingredients to a bowl, mix well, and then toss in sunflower seeds and black pepper if desired.

5. Add 1/4 the amount of mixed salad to each wrap in a line down the middle of the wrap, leaving about 3/4-inch from one end (we'll call this the bottom).

6. Use a spoon to generously dollop dressing on top of the salad. The avocado mix is really part dressing and part salad fixings so feel guilt-free and load it up if you like.

7. Fold the bottom end of the wrap up to meet the salad, and then fold each side over the salad. Enjoy!

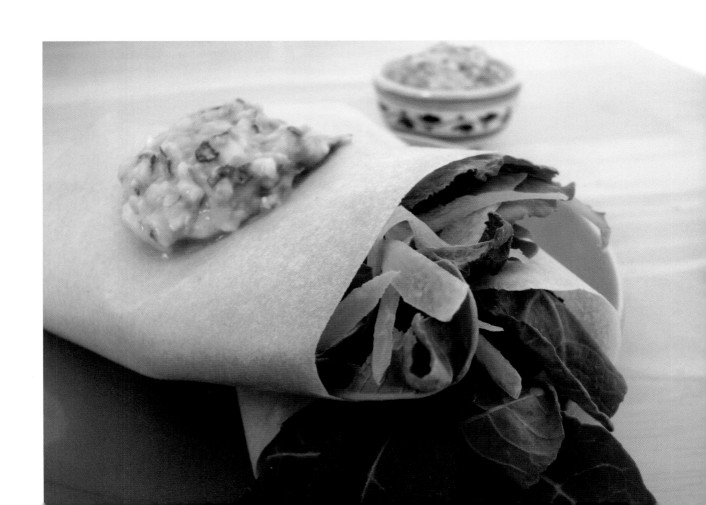

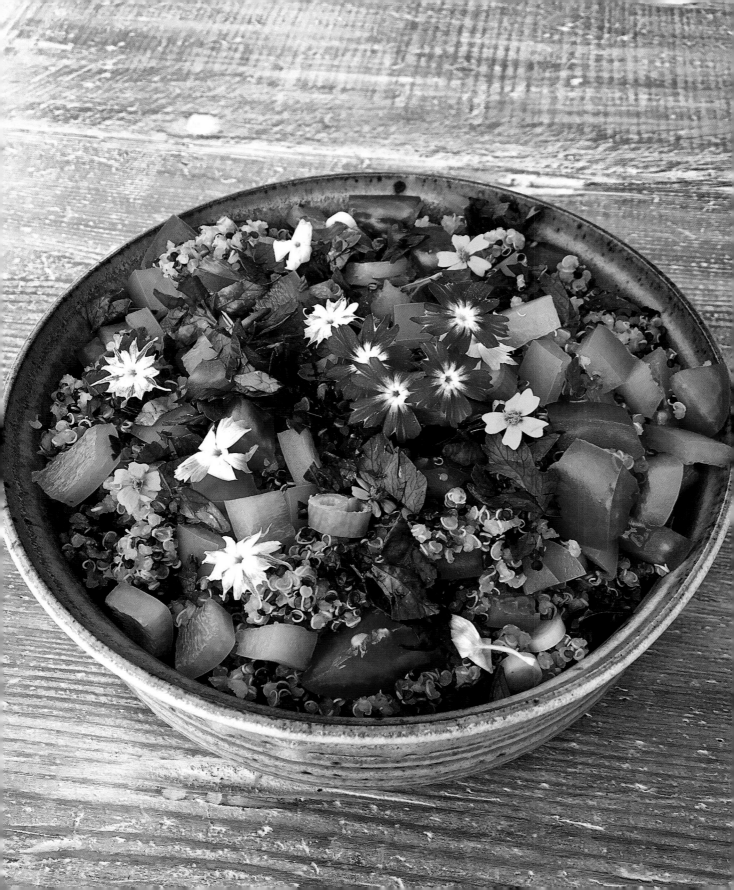

HEARTY VEGETARIAN

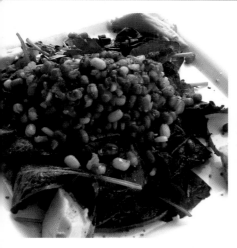
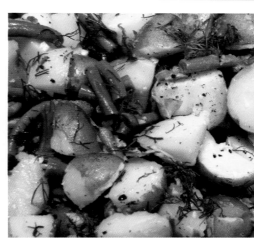
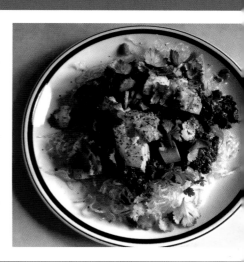

DISHES

FRITTATA

(GF, SF, DF, NF, VG)

Prep time: 20 minutes

Cook time: 10 minutes

Serves 2-plus as a full meal or 4 as a side dish

Ingredients

6 eggs

6 medium potatoes

1/2 Spanish onion

1 poblano pepper (optional)

EVOO

Salt and pepper to taste

Preparation

1. Thinly slice potatoes, and sauté in EVOO in an oven-proof frying pan until just tender—oven-proof pan needed only if broiling; see step four—otherwise, any large frying pan will do. Alternatively, boil potatoes until just tender, about ten minutes. Let cool then slice. This option is more hands-off but not quite as tasty.

2. Meanwhile, mix eggs in a bowl, and add chopped pepper, onion, salt, and pepper.

3. If sautéing potatoes, remove from pan with slotted spoon (leaving oil in pan), and stir into egg mixture. If boiling potatoes, stir them into egg mixture now.

4. Pour egg/potato mixture into frying pan, and cook over medium-low heat for about four to five minutes. At this point you can either flip and cook four minutes on other side or place oven-proof frying pan under a low broiler for about five minutes or until just brown. Serve while warm. This frittata is a meal on its own or is great with a side salad, veggie, or sprouted corn tortilla.

VEGETARIAN MACRO TRIO (MUNG BEANS, KALE, AVOCADO)

(GF, SF, DF, NF, VG, ED)

Total prep/cook time: 12–15 minutes

Serves 2 as a main dish or 4 as a side dish

A tasty vegetarian way to get some protein, carbohydrate, and fat.

Ingredients

    1 1/2 cups sprouted mung beans
      (truRoots is a good brand if you don't make your own
      sprouts)
    1 bunch of fresh kale or 1 box (~5 ounces) of
      Olivia's baby kale (or whatever brand you like)
    1 avocado
    4 cups of water
    EVOO
    Salt and pepper
    Fresh parsley for garnish, optional

Preparation

1. Bring water to a boil in a medium pot. Once boiling, add the sprouted mung beans and cook as directed on the package, or gently boil uncovered for five to seven minutes. Remove from heat, cover, and let sit for five to eight minutes until desired tenderness is reached. Once they are cooked to your liking, drain any excess water. If using homemade sprouted mung beans, steam them for two to five minutes or until desired tenderness.

2. While the mung beans are cooking, wash and chop the kale (if using fresh bunched), leaving a *small amount* of water on the leaves for cooking, or simply open the box of Olivia's and follow washing instructions on box (it is usually pre-washed), sprinkling with a *small amount* of water if not washing. In a large pot or skillet, heat kale on low and toss continually as it cooks for about five minutes. Alternatively, you can leave the kale raw and simply "tenderize" it by adding it to a large bowl, sprinkling with salt, and kneading it for three to five minutes until it softens and reduces in size. I tend to cook the kale in the fall/winter months and tenderize it during the spring and summer. Do whichever suits you.

3. Once the kale is ready, remove from heat and toss with EVOO (~1–2 TBSP), S&P to taste. Place on the bottom of a serving tray or individual plates.

4. Chop the avocado.

5. When the mung beans are ready, spoon the desired amount on top of the bed of kale. Top that with chopped pieces of avocado. Drizzle with EVOO and add more S&P if needed. Garnish with parsley if desired.

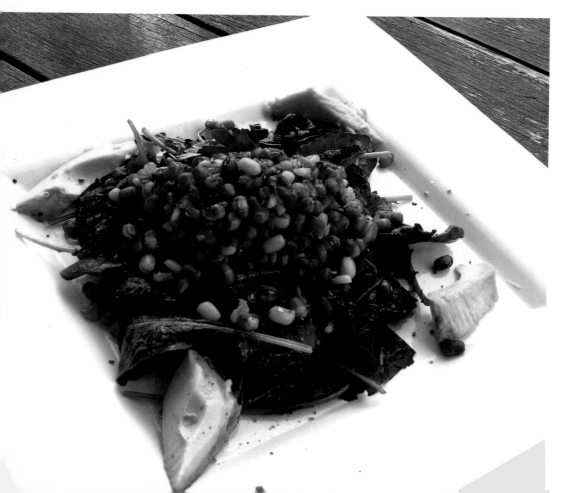

KELP NOODLE STIR-FRY

(GF, SF, DF, NF, VG)

Prep time: 10 minutes

Cook time: 10–15 minutes

Serves 4

Ingredients

1 package of kelp noodles, rinsed and drained
(I use ready-to-eat Gold Mine brand.)

1 large head of broccoli

20 mushrooms (shiitake, oyster, or baby bella are best)

3 tablespoon EVOO

2 garlic cloves, freshly chopped or pressed

2 teaspoons red pepper flakes

Salt to taste

Preparation

1. Divide rinsed kelp noodles into four servings and place on individual plates. You may need to use kitchen scissors to divide and cut the noodles.

2. Wash and chop mushrooms and broccoli. Set mushrooms aside and steam broccoli for 10–12 minutes or until tender. You can also boil broccoli for three minutes uncovered, and then immediately drain and remove from heat.

3. While the broccoli is cooking, heat EVOO in a pan on medium-low. When oil is hot, add garlic and red pepper flakes and sauté for 30 seconds. Add chopped mushrooms and continue to sauté until mushrooms are tender, about eight minutes. Once broccoli is done, place on top of noodles. Top with mushroom mixture.

4. Add S&P to taste. Drizzle with more EVOO if desired.

Note: I used broccoli and shiitake mushrooms, but you can choose one to three of your favorite vegetables (such as zucchini, peppers, tomato, eggplant, etc.)

DIJON KALE AND SQUASH

(GF, SF, DF, VG)

Prep time: 15 minutes to begin plus 15 minutes during cooking

Cook time: 30 minutes

Serves 4

Ingredients

1 bunch of kale (Or 1 box of baby kale. Olivia's is a reliable brand.)

1 butternut squash

1 teaspoon Dijon mustard

3 tablespoons balsamic vinegar

8 tablespoons EVOO

Salt and pepper to taste

3/4 cup chopped or ground almonds, optional

(I often use whole, skinless almonds after grinding them in a mortar and pestle because it's usually what I have in the house.)

Preparation

1. Preheat oven to 400°F. Peel and chop squash into half-inch cubes, toss with ~2 TBSP EVOO, salt, and pepper. Roast until tender for about 30 minutes. Stir the squash after 15 minutes. Once done, remove from oven and let cool slightly (five minutes).

2. Meanwhile, wash, chop, and spin dry the kale (stems removed) if using a fresh bunch, or do nothing if using Olivia's. Set aside. While the squash is cooking, whisk together 5 TBSP of EVOO, 3 TBSP vinegar, and 1 tsp. Dijon mustard in a small bowl. Season with S&P to taste (I use very little) and set aside.

3. There are two options for the kale. The first is to heat 1 TBSP EVOO in a pan and sauté the kale, tossing frequently, until it is just soft and still bright green (~two minutes over low to medium-low heat). The second option is to put raw kale in a bowl, sprinkle with salt (try to equally cover the kale with salt. It helps to put half the kale in the bowl, sprinkle with salt, and then add the rest and sprinkle again with salt). Knead the kale for three to five minutes (again, it depends on type of kale) or until it reduces in volume and becomes soft.

No cooking necessary. I usually go with the first option in the cooler months and the second in the warmer weather.

4. When the kale is done, toss with 3–4 TBSP of the mustard dressing and transfer to serving dish. Add the squash and almonds and toss gently. Season with S&P if needed. Use the remaining dressing if desired.

Notes: This recipe can be made nut-free by omitting the almonds. If you want the added protein, add the almonds. Sesame seeds and sunflower seeds make good substitutes for the almonds. Additionally, shaved Parmesan cheese makes a nice, but unnecessary, garnish and is optional. Note that the recipe will no longer be dairy-free if you add the cheese.

To make a meal out of this dish, serve it rolled in a paleo coconut wrap (see resources). Delicious and filling!

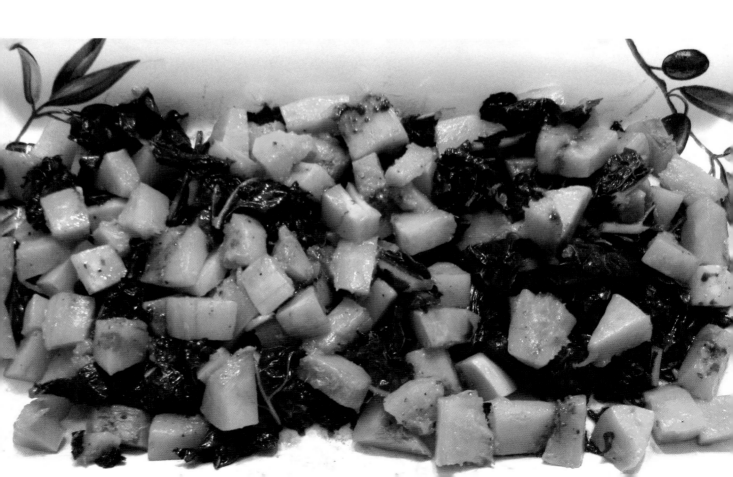

SPICED VEGETABLE STEW

(GF, SF, DF, NF*, VG)

Prep time: 15 minutes

Cook time: 20 minutes

Serves 4–6

This dish can be made using only some of the veggies listed. I have made it with only carrots and sweet potatoes, and it comes out just as delicious. The gist is to use two to three vegetables and these spices.

Ingredients

1/3 cup coconut oil
  (or use EVOO to be purely nut-free)*
1 small onion
2 garlic cloves, pressed or finely chopped
1 teaspoon ground cumin
1 teaspoon turmeric
1 teaspoon paprika
1/2 teaspoon cinnamon
1/2 teaspoon cayenne
1/2 teaspoon salt
pinch of saffron
1 cup carrots, sliced into small pieces
  (the smaller you chop them, the faster they cook)
4 cups sweet potatoes
  (2–3 medium or large sweet potatoes) or butternut squash, cubed
1 cup eggplant, cubed
  (zucchini can also be used and should be if eliminating nightshades)
1 cup cooked garbanzo beans
1/4 cup fresh parsley, chopped

Preparation

1. In a large stew pot, heat the coconut oil and sauté the onion for two to three minutes. Add the garlic and spices (except the salt and saffron), stirring continuously.

2. Add the vegetables in the order listed above, cooking each for a few minutes (two to five), or until its color deepens, before adding the next one. Add salt with the last vegetable, and cook for about two minutes more.

3. Add the garbanzo beans and saffron.

4. There should be some liquid at the bottom of the pot from the vegetables, but if not, add about 1/3 cup of water. Cover the stew and simmer on low until the vegetables are tender, about 10–15 minutes. The carrots usually take the longest, so once they are tender the stew is ready.

5. Add the chopped parsley on top once you've plated the stew.

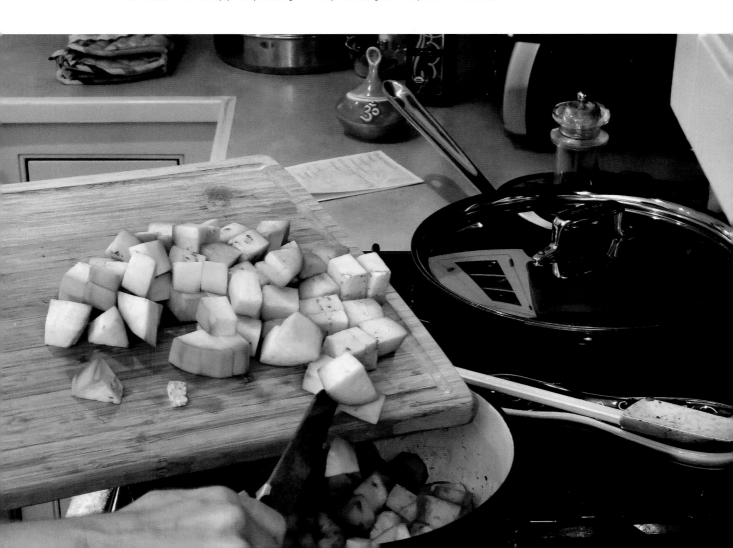

QUINOA WITH GREENS

(GF, SF, DF, NF, VG, ED)

Prep time: 2 minutes

Cook time: 20 minutes

Serves 4 as a side dish or 2 as a meal

Ingredients

1 cup quinoa, rinsed

2 cups water or broth

2 1/2 ounces (half of a 5 oz. box) of Olivia's greens (or your favorite greens)

2-4 tablespoons EVOO

Salt and pepper to taste

Preparation

1. Place quinoa and water or broth in a medium saucepan and bring to a boil.

2. Reduce to a simmer, cover, and cook until liquid is absorbed, about 20 minutes.

3. Once quinoa is cooked, stir in your choice of raw greens such as spinach, Swiss chard, or kale. The hot quinoa will cook the greens just enough.

4. Add S&P to taste and drizzle with EVOO.

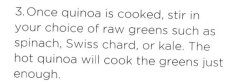

Serving Suggestion: This dish makes a great stuffing for a bell pepper (see recipe on page 85).

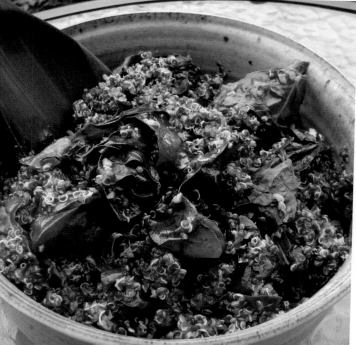

SAFFRON RICE

(GF, SF, DF*, NF, VG)

Prep time: 10 minutes hands-off

Cook time: 20 minutes (some hands on)

Serves 6

Ingredients

    1 pinch of saffron

    1 1/2 cups basmati rice

    3 tablespoon unsalted butter (or ghee)

    4 bay leaves

    7 bits of cinnamon bark

      (Don't substitute with ground cinnamon, as it will take over.)

    7 whole cloves (can use 1/4 tsp. ground cloves but whole cloves recommended)

    1/2 teaspoon salt

    7 whole cardamom pods (or ~25 seeds or 1/2 tsp. powder)

    4 cups + 1 tablespoon hot water

Preparation

1. Soak the saffron in 1 TBSP water for ten minutes.

2. Rinse rice.

3. Heat a pot over medium heat, and add butter or ghee.

4. Add bay leaves, cinnamon, cloves, salt, and cardamom, and mix well for ~one minute.

5. Turn heat to low, add rice and stir well, sautéing for about two minutes.

6. Pour in the 4 cups of hot water and saffron and bring to a gentle boil. Boil uncovered for five minutes.

7. Turn down heat to medium and boil, partially covered, for five minutes, stirring twice to prevent sticking.

8. Turn heat to low, fully cover and simmer for ten minutes or until tender.

Tip: If you don't have time to stand at the stove during steps six and seven, then follow steps one through five, add water and cook as directed on bag of rice. If you use brown basmati rice, it will take an extra five to ten minutes to cook.

*This recipe may be ok for you if you tolerate butter or ghee.

. . . .

Serving Suggestion: This dish makes a great stuffing for a bell pepper (see recipe on page 85).

. . . .

FRESH POTATO SALAD WITH GREEN BEANS

(GF, SF, DF, VG, NF*)

Prep time: 15 minutes

Cook time: 20 minutes

Serves 4

Ingredients

28 ounces small potatoes (any kind)

8 ounces fresh green beans

2 cloves of garlic

Large handful of fresh herbs

(such as basil, dill, flat parsley, thyme, lemon thyme, or rosemary)

2–3 tablespoons apple cider vinegar (depending on your taste)

1/4 cup EVOO

Salt and pepper to taste

2 tablespoons pine nuts (optional)

* Nut-free if you leave the pine nuts out.

Preparation

1. Wash potatoes and boil in large pot of water for 15–20 minutes depending on size of potatoes. Do not overcook or they will be mushy.

2. While potatoes are cooking, wash and chop green beans into ~1-inch pieces. Steam for ~eight minutes or until just tender. Do not overcook.

3. Once you have beans cooking, wash and chop basil and/or other herbs.

4. When potatoes are done, remove them from pot and allow them to cool a few minutes. When cool enough to handle, quarter them (chop into bite-size pieces) and add to serving bowl.

5. When green beans are done, add to potatoes.

6. Press garlic into potatoes and green beans, add chopped herbs, EVOO, vinegar, and S&P.

7. Stir well, and add more EVOO if needed since potatoes may absorb it.

Notes: This dish can be served immediately or made up to one day ahead. Asparagus can be used in place of green beans.

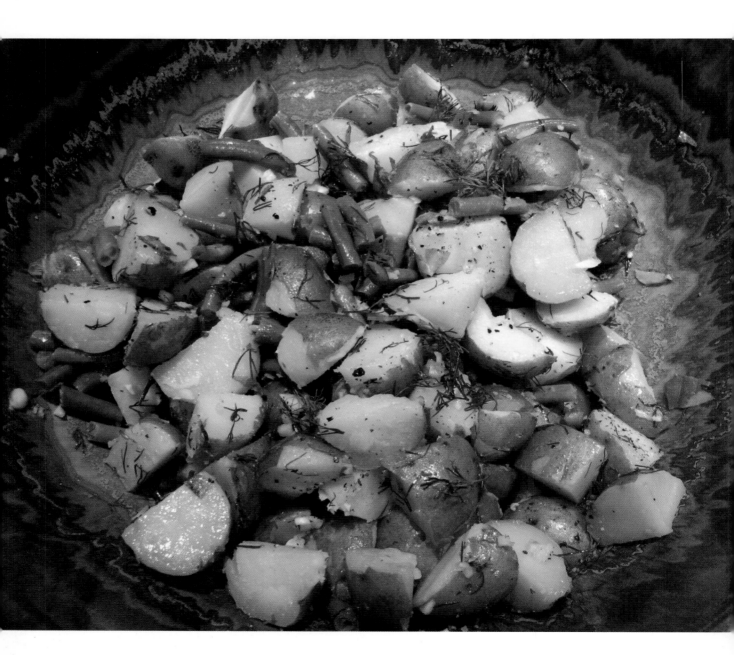

SAGE POTATOES

(GF, SF, DF, NF, VG, ED)

Prep time: 5 minutes

Cook time: 10 minutes plus 15–20 minutes

Serves: 4

Ingredients

    10 small–medium red potatoes or 4 medium sweet potatoes

    1 large bunch of sage (~20 large leaves)

    2 large garlic cloves

    Pinch of lavender, optional

    1/4 cup EVOO

    1 teaspoon black pepper

    1 teaspoon salt

Preparation

1. Scrub potatoes then boil them for ten minutes. Preheat oven to 375°F.

2. While potatoes are boiling, put all other ingredients in a chopper or blender and blend thoroughly. You can blend lavender or leave whole and sprinkle on top.

3. Remove potatoes from water and cut in half or into 1–2-inch pieces depending upon how large the potatoes are and your preference. Place in a glass baking dish and cover with sage mixture. Bake at 375°F 15–20 minutes or until done.

   Tip: Double the amount of sage mixture and use on chicken to make an easy meal out of it. Serve with sautéed greens.

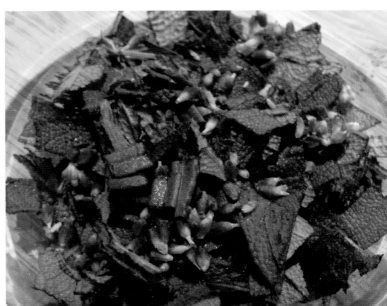

SPICED QUINOA SALAD

(GF, SF, DF, NF, VG, ED)

Prep/cook time: 30 minutes

(Most of the prep can be done while the quinoa is cooking.)

Serves 2 as a meal or 4 as a side dish

Ingredients

1 cup quinoa, rinsed

2 cups liquid (broth or water)

1–2 bell peppers, preferably orange for color

1 chili pepper (optional)

1 box of cherry tomatoes

1 small cucumber (optional)

1 bunch of scallions (can also use half a red onion)

1/3 bunch of parsley (1/2–1 cup)

1 teaspoon ground cumin*

1 teaspoon ground coriander*

1 teaspoon turmeric*

1/2 teaspoon cayenne pepper*

Salt and pepper to taste

EVOO and/or butter

* These are the spices I use, but you can use your favorite spices here.

Preparation

1. Prepare quinoa as directed on package or as follows. Use 1 cup quinoa to 2 cups liquid (broth or water). Bring to a boil then cover and simmer for 20 minutes or until liquid is absorbed. For added flavor you can sauté the quinoa in EVOO or butter for three to five minutes before adding the liquid. Add spices, salt, and pepper when you add the liquid. If using unground spices such as cumin seeds, sauté them in EVOO or butter before sautéing the quinoa (also see optional preparation below).

2. While the quinoa is cooking, chop all vegetables and parsley into bite-size pieces.

3. Once quinoa is cooked, scoop it into a large bowl and let cool slightly.

4. Drizzle with EVOO (~2 TBSP), and add the chopped vegetables and parsley.

5. Stir well and serve.

This dish is delicious warm or room temperature, which makes it great for parties or making a few hours ahead of time.

• •

Serving Suggestion: This dish makes a great stuffing for a bell pepper (see recipe on page 85). If using to stuff a pepper, leave the bell pepper out of this recipe.

• •

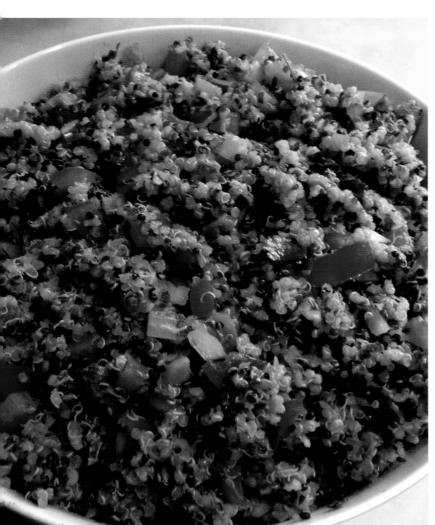

Optional preparation

(my favorite method)

This variation takes an additional five minutes but gives the dish more of a curry flavor. The only additional ingredient used is 1 teaspoon of cumin seeds, but you can leave it out if you don't have any.

Heat butter or EVOO in pot on low. Add cumin seeds and sauté until just brown (~one minute). Add all other spices and sauté another minute. Add quinoa and stir until coated with spices, and then continue to sauté an additional minute or two. Add liquid, bring to a boil, and then cover and simmer for 15–20 minutes or until liquid is absorbed. Proceed from step two above.

PESTO RISOTTO

(GF, SF, VG*)

Prep time: 15 minutes

Cook time: 20 minutes (hands on)

Serves 2 as a meal or 4 as a side dish

Ingredients

For the risotto

1 1/2 cups Arborio rice

4–5 cups stock (chicken or vegetable for vegetarian)*

1/2 Spanish onion (or 1 small Spanish onion), finely chopped

3 tablespoons (1/4 cup) unsalted butter

1/2 cup dry white wine**

1/2 cup freshly grated Parmesan cheese

Salt and pepper to taste

**Don't skimp on the quality of wine used. Use a decent bottle of wine, as you will taste it.

For the pesto

1 bunch (16 oz.) of fresh basil, stemmed

1/4 cup fresh parsley (optional)

2–3 cloves of garlic, peeled

  (Depending on how garlicky you like it. I use three.)

1/4 cup pine nuts (optional)

1/3 cup EVOO

Salt and pepper to taste

Preparation

1. Place all of the pesto ingredients in a chopper or blender, holding back half the EVOO. Blend to a smooth consistency. Set aside.

2. Pour broth into a pot, and bring to just below boiling. Turn heat to simmer, and keep the broth warm while cooking the risotto. Keep a large ladle nearby.

3. In a large, heavy-bottomed pot, melt butter over medium heat then add onion and sauté until onion is soft—about two to three minutes.

4. Add Arborio rice to the pot and stir until it's covered in butter, and then pour in the wine.

5. Once the wine has almost all evaporated, begin adding the simmering broth one ladle full at a time (1/2 cup at a time), stirring continuously. Each time the broth becomes absorbed, add more. Stir regularly and continue with this process until the rice is tender (but al dente), about 20 minutes.

6. Once the risotto i*s al dente*, remove from heat and stir in the grated Parmesan cheese. Add S&P to taste.

7. Scoop risotto into a serving dish, and stir in the pesto.

Note: This recipe can be made nut-free if you leave the pine nuts out.

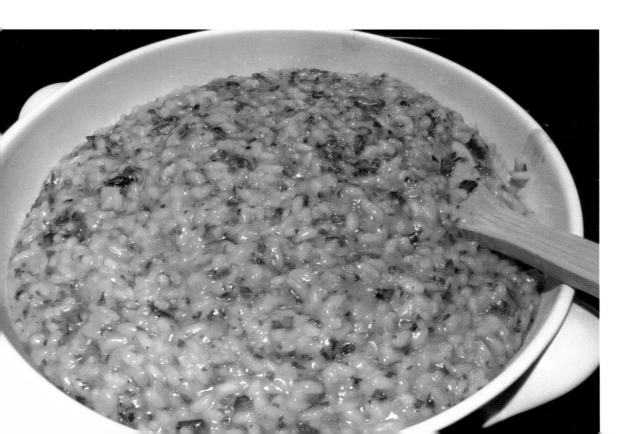

MUNG DAL KHICHADI

(GF, SF, DF*, NF, VG, ED*)

Prep time: 15 minutes

Cook time: 15–20 minutes

Serves 2 as a meal or 4 as a side dish

Ingredients

1 cup basmati rice**

1 cup mung dal***

6 cloves of garlic

1/2-inch piece of fresh ginger

1 teaspoon cumin seeds

1/2 teaspoon turmeric powder

1/2 teaspoon coriander powder

1 small green chili (optional)

1–2 tablespoon ghee or unsalted butter

Salt to taste

Water (~2–4 cups)

* This recipe may be ok for you if you tolerate butter or ghee.

** If using brown basmati, note that it takes slightly longer to cook than white.

*** If using whole mung dal, soak it for as long as possible (1-8 hours) before cooking. For ease, I use sprouted mung beans from trüRoots, which do not need to be soaked at all.

Preparation

1. Prepare rice and mung dal by rinsing, soaking, and measuring as necessary, and then set aside.

2. Finely chop ginger, garlic, and chili.

3. Heat ghee or butter in pressure cooker or pot, then add cumin seeds and fry until just brown.

4. Add ginger, garlic, and chili. Stir.

5. Add turmeric, coriander, and salt. Stir well.

6. Add rice and mung dal. Mix well with spices.

7. Add enough water to cover the mung dal and rice so that there is 1/4-inch of water on top of it all if using a pressure cooker, and add another 1/2 cup of water on top of that if using a regular pot.

8. If using a pressure cooker, cook on medium-high until the first whistle, then turn to low heat for another five to seven minutes or until rice and mung dal are just soft (overcooking will cause the mung dal to be mushy). If using a regular covered pot, bring to just before boiling, then turn to low and simmer for 10–15 minutes or until soft.

Khichadi is a staple in Ayurvedic cooking and consists of mung dal, basmati rice, and specific spices to create a balanced, easily digested meal. The proportions are usually one part dal to two parts rice but can be varied along with the spices depending upon the healing need. The following recipe is adapted from Zanjabee Integrative Medicine & Primary Care, and is a simple khichadi that provides the right amount of comfort and nourishment to just about everyone.

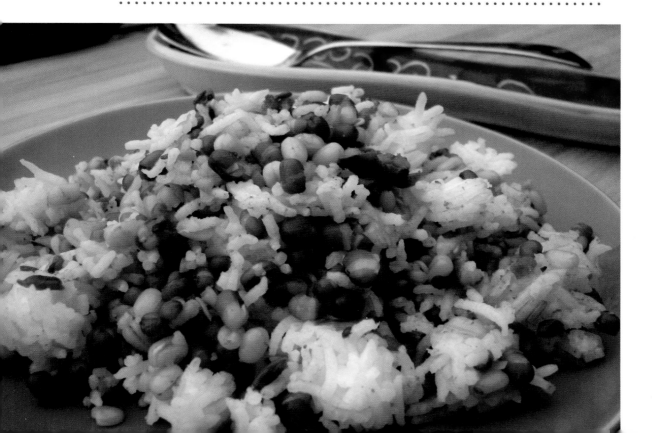

RED LENTILS WITH RICE

(ADAPTED FROM *AYURVEDIC COOKING FOR SELF-HEALING* BY USHA LAD AND DR. VASANT LAD)

(GF, SF, DF*, NF, VG, ED)

Total prep/cook time: 30 minutes (much prep is done during cooking)

Serves 2–4 (meal or side dish)

Ingredients

- 1 cup split red lentils, rinsed (can also use soaked whole red lentils)**
- 1 cup of rice
- 4 1/2 cups water
- 2 teaspoon ghee, unsalted butter, or EVOO if dairy-free*
- 1 teaspoon cumin seeds
- 1 teaspoon black mustard seeds
- 2 large cloves of garlic, chopped
- 5 curry leaves, fresh or dried
- 1 handful of cilantro leaves, chopped
- 1/2 teaspoon turmeric
- 1/4 teaspoon ground cloves
- 1/4 teaspoon ground cardamom
- 1/4 teaspoon black pepper
- 1 large bay leaf
- 1/4 teaspoon cinnamon
- 1/4 teaspoon cayenne pepper
- 1/2 teaspoon salt

** I use split red lentils because they don't require soaking, though you can soak for an hour if desired, and they cook quickly compared to whole lentils. If you use whole red lentils, soak overnight if possible or at least four hours, rinse, drain, and adjust cooking time accordingly, checking for doneness. Cooking time will depend on how long you soaked the lentils; the longer you soak, the less the cooking time. If you soak split red lentils the cooking time is closer to five to ten minutes.

Preparation

1. Add rice to 2 cups of boiling water (or cook as directed on rice package). White basmati rice usually takes 20–25 minutes to cook. See package for details.

2. Chop garlic and cilantro.

3. In a separate pot from the rice, add lentils to 2 1/2 cups of water and bring to a boil. Reduce to medium-low heat and simmer uncovered for 12–15 minutes** or until tender. Gently stir a few times during cooking to prevent them from sticking, but do not over-stir.

4. While lentils are cooking, heat ghee, butter, or oil in a small frying pan over low-medium heat, and then add mustard seeds and cumin seeds, stirring frequently. When the seeds make a popping sound, stir in the garlic and brown *slightly.*

5. Add the curry leaves, cilantro, turmeric, cloves, cardamom, black pepper, bay leaf, cinnamon and cayenne. Mix quickly. Add a small amount of water (between a tsp. and a TBSP) to help the spices mix well.

6. If you want your lentils to be a bit soupy, add water to desired consistency. If you want them to be dry, drain water from lentils to desired consistency.

7. Stir the spice mixture into the pot of lentils and mix well.

8. Bring to a gentle boil for one to two minutes. Serve over rice.

Note: These lentils can be served dry as a side dish instead of over rice.

BUCKWHEAT NOODLES IN GINGER GARLIC SAUCE

(GF, SF, DF, NF*, VG, ED*)

Prep time: 10 minutes

Cook time: 5–10 minutes

Serves 2 as a meal with side salad or veggie or 4 as a side dish

Ingredients

8-ounce package of buckwheat noodles

(See resources for recommended brands. Be sure there is no wheat flour mixed in if you are wheat or gluten-free.)

2–3-inch piece of fresh ginger

2 cloves garlic

3 tablespoons coconut oil

1/2 teaspoon ground cumin

1/2 teaspoon ground coriander

Sprig of fresh dill or 1 teaspoon dried dill

1/2 teaspoon gharam masala (optional)**

2 teaspoons coconut vinegar (optional)

Salt and pepper to taste

Preparation

1. Get a pot of water boiling for the noodles while you peel and chop ginger and garlic.

2. Add noodles to boiling water and cook for ~five minutes or as stated on package.

3. Meanwhile, add coconut oil to a frying pan and sauté the spices, including black pepper, for one minute. Add the ginger, garlic, and salt, and sauté until just golden.

4. Once noodles are cooked, rinse in cold water if necessary (see package instructions) and toss in frying pan with sauce. Serve immediately. Garnish with dill.

*Use other oil, such as EVOO, for nut-free.

**If you don't have gharam masala, you can add 1/4 teaspoon each of cloves, coriander, and cinnamon.

Note: I did not intentionally add coconut vinegar the first time I made this recipe, but I served the noodles with a side salad that was dressed with coconut oil and coconut vinegar. A bit of the vinegar made its way into my noodles, and I enjoyed the flavor. Try the noodles with or without the vinegar (avoid it if nut-free is desired). Serve noodles with a salad and/or zucchini, Indian style (page 88).

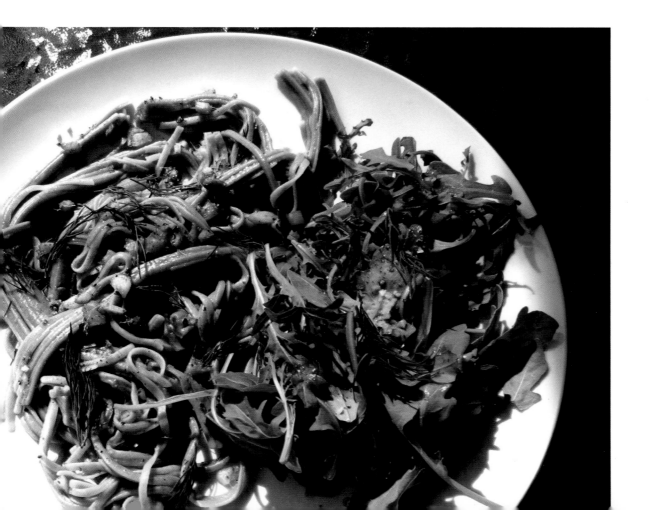

RAW KELP NOODLE SALAD

(GF, SF, DF, NF, VG)

Prep time: 10–15 minutes

Cook time: 0 minutes

Serves: 2

Ingredients

3 large kale leaves

2 lettuce leaves

Handful of cilantro leaves

Juice of half a lemon

5 ounces kelp noodles (see resources)

Half an avocado

1/4 of a cucumber

1 teaspoon sesame seeds

1 teaspoon dulse flakes (optional, see resources)

Salt and pepper

Hot sesame oil, regular sesame oil, or EVOO for drizzling

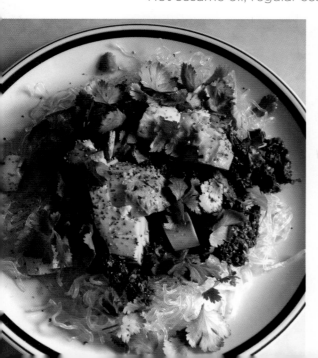

Preparation

1. Rinse kale, lettuce, and cilantro. Add to a chopper or blender with the lemon juice and roughly chop.

2. Rinse and drain kelp noodles. Cut them if desired and plate them.

3. Slice avocado and cucumber.

4. Scoop kale mixture over the noodles. Put avocado and cucumber on top. Sprinkle with sesame seeds, dulse, and S&P to taste. Drizzle hot sesame oil on top sparingly.

Note: This meal is great for raw vegetarians but can be difficult to digest for someone not used to eating a lot of raw food. If the latter category describes you, try this meal in small portions.

SOUPS

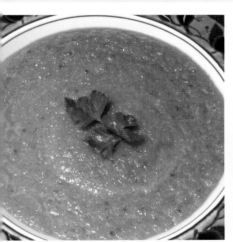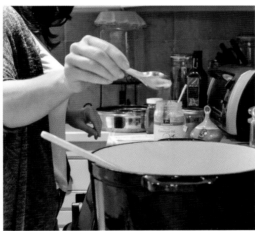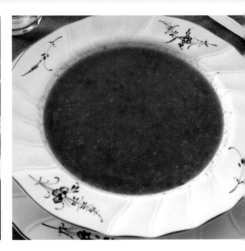

MUSHROOM SOUP

(GF, SF, DF, NF, VG, ED)

This recipe is a family favorite, handed down by my mother.

Prep time: 40 minutes, including initial sautéing

Cook time: 30 minutes

Serves 4–6

Ingredients

3/4 pound mushrooms (crimini and baby bella work best)

48 ounces of mushroom broth

(see references for brand name and where to buy)

2 cloves garlic

1 small onion

1 tomato (can use canned crushed tomato)

2 tablespoons fresh parsley or 1/2 teaspoon dried parsley

1 small potato (Yukon is best), optional

(adds thickness, but I often leave it out)

1/4 cup EVOO

Salt and pepper to taste

1–2 teaspoons herbs de Provence (or oregano, thyme, rosemary, or marjoram)

Preparation

1. Clean and slice mushrooms, set aside.

2. Chop onion, tomato if fresh, and parsley, set aside.

3. Peel and dice potato, if using, and set aside.

4. In a large pot sauté mushrooms, garlic (use garlic press and press it directly into pan), and onion in 1/4 cup EVOO.

5. When above veggies are soft (~ten minutes), add broth, tomato, potato, parsley, pepper, and herbs de Provence (other desired herbs) to the pot.

6. Cover pot, bring to a boil, and then simmer on low until potato is soft, about 15–20 minutes (simmer 10–15 minutes if not using potato).

7. Let cool five to ten minutes, just enough to safely handle it for step eight.

8. Add soup to a blender to purée, in multiple batches if necessary. You can purée all of the soup or leave about 1 cup behind so some pieces of mushroom remain (try to purée all of the potato).

9. Can be made up to one day ahead.

Notes: You can also use chicken, vegetable, or beef broth, but choose mushroom or vegetable broth for a vegetarian recipe. I usually throw in a few shiitake for their added health benefit and wonderful flavor.

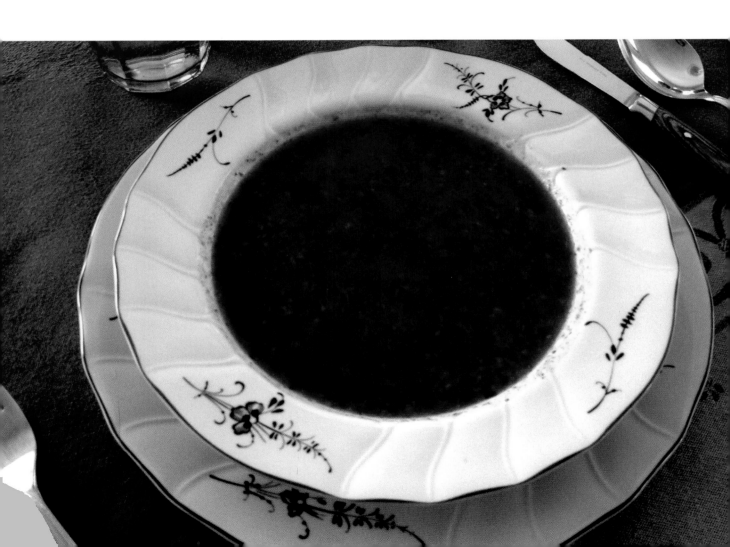

CARROT GINGER SOUP

(GF, SF, DF*, VG)

Total prep/cook time: 30 minutes

Serves 4

Ingredients

- 1 1/2 pounds of carrots
- 3–4 cups of water (depending on how thick you like it)
- 1 clove garlic
- 3–4 tablespoons of fresh ginger (according to taste)
- 1/2 an onion (optional)
- 1–2 tablespoons butter or coconut oil*
  (use butter for nut-free and coconut oil for dairy-free)
- 1/2 teaspoon ground cumin
- 1/2 teaspoon ground fennel
- 1/4 teaspoon cinnamon
- 1/4 teaspoon nutmeg
- 1/4 teaspoon cloves
- 1 teaspoon salt
- Juice from 1/2 a lemon
- 1/2 cup of your favorite nuts or seeds (optional)
  (cashews, sesame seeds, or sunflower seeds go well)*
- Fresh cilantro for garnish (can also use parsley or dill)

*Use butter and omit nuts if you desire a nut-free recipe. I usually make this without the nuts, and it's delicious.

Feel free to play around with the spices listed according to your taste.

Tip: I get a variety of orange, yellow, and purple carrots from a local farmer, which makes for a deliciously colorful soup.

Preparation

1. Scrub or peel carrots and chop into 1-inch pieces. Add carrots and water to a pot, cover, and bring to a boil. Once boiling, turn down to a simmer and cook until carrots are tender, about 10–15 minutes. Let carrots/water cool just enough to safely add them to a blender or Vitamix.

2. While carrots cook, peel and chop onion, ginger, and garlic. Heat butter or coconut oil in a small pot or skillet and sauté onions, if using, for about three minutes. Add garlic, ginger, salt, and spices and sauté on low heat for about five minutes more or until onion is cooked. Stir in lemon juice.

3. Add carrots in their water, plus the spiced ginger mix, to a blender or Vitamix. Also add nuts or seeds if using. Blend briefly, in batches if necessary, to a thick purée or your desired texture. You can always add more water, a little at a time, as you're blending if it's too thick, then reheat if necessary.

4. Garnish with cilantro.

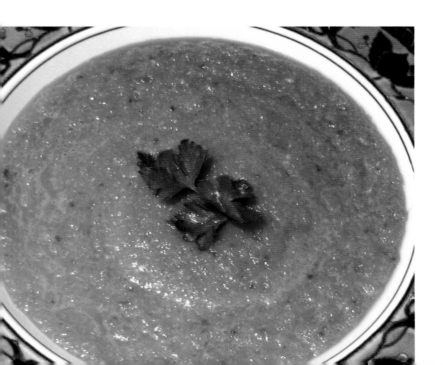

BUTTERNUT SQUASH SOUP

(GF, SF, DF, NF, VG, ED)

Prep time: 5 minutes

Cook time: 90 minutes

Serves: 4

Ingredients

1 large butternut squash

1–2 cloves of garlic

3 tablespoons EVOO

1 teaspoon red pepper flakes

4 cups of water or broth

1 cinnamon stick

Salt to taste

I love how light this soup is.

Preparation

1. Preheat oven to 350°F. Slice squash in half, and remove seeds. Roast squash until tender, about 40-45 minutes.

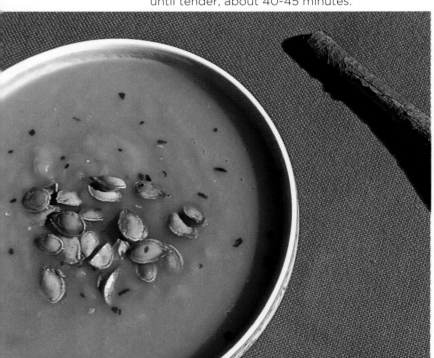

2. Once squash is cooked, scoop it out of skin and add to a blender to purée.

3. Chop garlic. Heat EVOO in a soup pot, and add garlic and red pepper flakes. Sauté about one minute. Add the squash purée, cinnamon stick, and water or broth.

4. Simmer for 30–45 minutes. Serve warm.

LUCKY LENTIL SOUP

(GF, SF, DF, NF, VG*, ED)

Prep time: 20 minutes

Cook time: 1 hour

Serves: 4

Ingredients

1 1/2 cups lentils
(I use brown lentils for this recipe. You can also use split peas.)

1/2 pound carrots (~2 or 3 large carrots)

1 onion

3 cloves of garlic

48 ounces chicken or vegetable broth*

1 bay leaf

1/4 teaspoon celery seeds

1/4–1/2 cup fresh parsley (or ~1 TBSP dry), plus extra for garnish

1 teaspoon of cumin powder or seeds (optional)

EVOO for sautéing vegetables

Salt and pepper to taste

Preparation

1. Peel and chop carrots, garlic, and onion.

2. In a large soup pot, sauté carrots, garlic, onion, and cumin in EVOO until onion is soft.

3. Meanwhile, rinse lentils in hot water until water runs clear (about two full rinses).

4. When onion is just soft, add broth, lentils, bay leaf, parsley, celery seeds, salt, and pepper.

5. Simmer with lid on for about one hour. If you prefer a thicker soup, remove 2–3 cups once cooked, blend, and then add back into the remaining soup. Garnish with parsley.

*I like the flavor better with chicken broth, but use vegetable broth for a vegetarian option.

Note: If you know you're going to make lentil soup ahead of time, soak the lentils in filtered water for one to eight hours, and then rinse as instructed above.

· ·

When I was a kid, my grandmother used to tell me that lentils were chocolate chips in order to get me to eat more soup. It worked. I didn't mind lentil soup, but I just didn't eat enough to please the Sicilian in her. Every New Year's Day, it is a tradition in my mother's house to eat lentil soup. Lentil soup is eaten on New Year's Day in several cultures. The coin-shaped lentils are thought to represent prosperity. It's a warm and delicious tradition to ring in the New Year with family and friends. And of course, it's warm and delicious any time of year. May you have peace and prosperity.

· ·

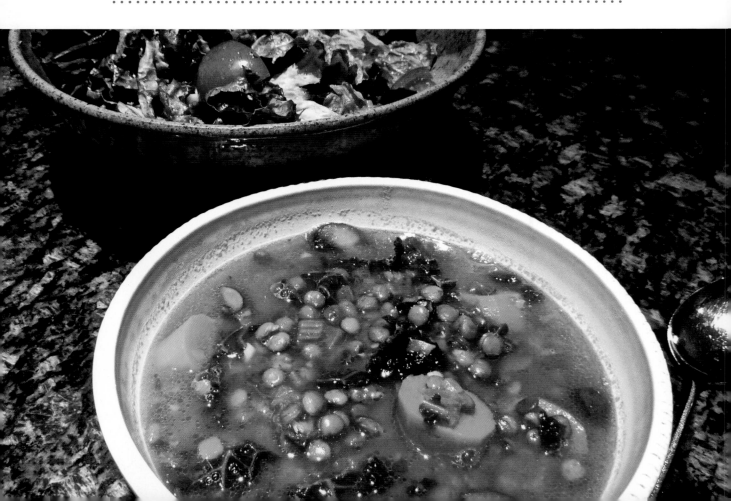

SAUCES

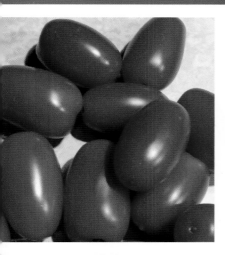
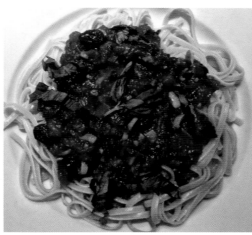
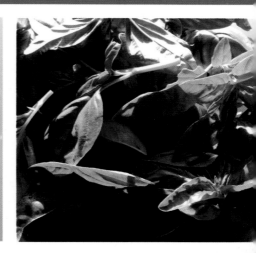

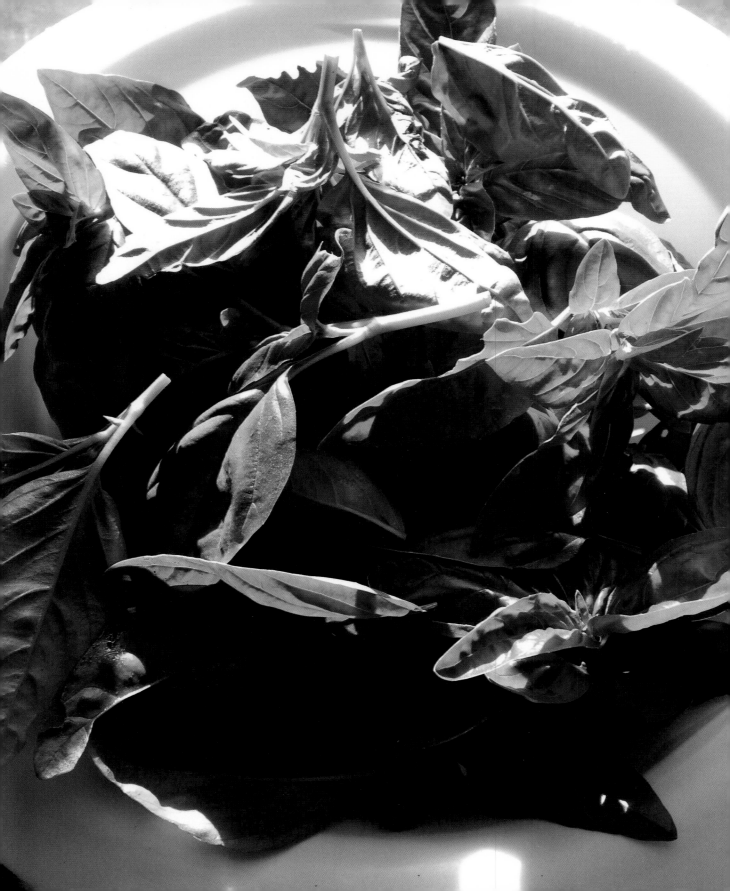

PESTO

(GF, SF, VG)

Prep time: 15 minutes

Cook time: 0

Serves 4

Ingredients

1 large bunch of fresh basil (~2 packed cups), stemmed

1/4 cup fresh parsley, (optional)

2–3 cloves of garlic, peeled

1/4 cup pine nuts (omit to make nut-free)

1/2 cup Parmesan cheese, plus more to taste (freshly grated is best)*

1/4–1/3 cup EVOO*

1/2 teaspoon each of salt and pepper, plus more to taste

Preparation

1. Add basil, parsley, garlic, pine nuts, S&P, and half the amount of EVOO to a blender or chopper. You may need to add everything in multiple batches if using a small chopper. Blend or pulse until smooth or desired texture is reached.

2. Test it and add S&P to taste. Add more EVOO as needed to achieve desired texture. Pulse or gently blend again to incorporate S&P and EVOO.

3. Scoop pesto into a bowl, and stir in the Parmesan cheese.

4. Spoon over pasta, polenta, fish, chicken, beef, or anything you desire. If using on a vegetable or carbohydrate of any kind you can drizzle with the remaining EVOO and cheese.

* If using pesto on meat (especially fish or beef), I recommend leaving out the cheese. If using on chicken or beef you can omit the extra drizzle of EVOO at the end. This recipe can be made dairy-free by omitting the cheese and/or nut-free by omitting the pine nuts—it will still taste delicious.

Sicilian pesto—add a large handful (1/2 box) of cherry tomatoes and 1 teaspoon of crushed red pepper flakes to the above ingredients, and then substitute almonds for pine nuts and you have Sicilian pesto.

CHIMICHURRI

(GF, SF, DF, NF, VG, ED)

Prep time: 10 minutes

Serves 2-plus

Ingredients

- 1 packed cup of fresh cilantro
- 1/2 packed cup fresh parsley
- 2 cloves of garlic
- 1 teaspoon crushed red pepper flakes
- 1 teaspoon oregano
- 3 tablespoons red wine vinegar (can use lemon juice instead if you prefer)
- 1/3 cup EVOO
- Salt and pepper to taste

Preparation

1. Add all ingredients except S&P to a chopper or blender and gently blend until mixed.

2. Add S&P to taste.

Notes: Use chimichuri as a marinade or sauce for meat or fish. Can be used right away or made several hours, up to one day, ahead of time.

FRESH TOMATO SAUCE

(GF, SF, DF, NF, VG, ED)

Prep time: 15 minutes

Cook time: 0–2 hours, depending on your preference

Serves 4

Ingredients

> 6 fresh tomatoes, quartered
>
> 1/2 bunch fresh basil
>
> 1 tablespoon dried or fresh oregano
>
> 1/4 cup EVOO
>
> Salt and pepper to taste

Preparation

1. Put all ingredients in a Vitamix and blend on high until puréed and well mixed, up to two minutes.

2. Sauce can be served as is, semi-raw, or simmered in a pot on the stove for up to two hours.

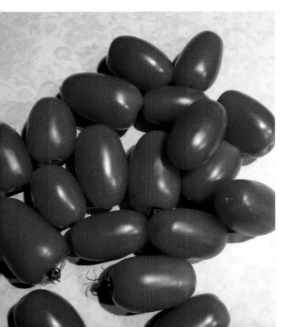

Note: If you blend for only a few minutes, your sauce will be on the raw side and need to be heated on the stove for a traditional tomato sauce. Alternatively, you can blend all ingredients until heat is created (you'll see some steam form and feel a bit of heat on the outside of the Vitamix), and this will cook the sauce. Once you feel heat, you can continue to blend another minute or so. Cooking the sauce completely in the Vitamix (no stove) takes three to five minutes. The sauce may be orange and almost creamy in texture from the mixing as opposed to the usual red, "chunky" looking sauce when the stove is used. I prefer the stove when I have time and use the Vitamix when time is limited.

Tip: If heating the sauce on the stove, you can add raw meatballs and cook them in the sauce as it simmers.

PUTTANESCA

(GF, SF, DF, NF, ED)

Prep time: 10 minutes

Cook time: 20 minutes

Serves 4

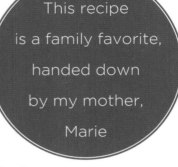

This recipe is a family favorite, handed down by my mother, Marie

Ingredients

4 cloves of garlic

1 small onion (optional)

1 can (~14 ounces) of San Marzano tomatoes or 6 large fresh tomatoes when in season

4 teaspoons of tomato paste (needed only if using fresh tomatoes)

1/2–1 teaspoon of red pepper flakes

3–4 teaspoons anchovy paste or 1 can of anchovies

1/3 cup Kalamata olives

1–2 tablespoon capers

Handful of fresh basil or parsley (plus more for garnish if desired)

Preparation

1. Chop onion, garlic, olives, tomatoes if using fresh, and anchovies if using instead of paste.

2. Sauté onion and garlic for one minute. When onion is just beginning to get soft, add anchovies or anchovy paste and tomato paste if using. Stir until anchovies are soft and well incorporated into the mix.

3. Add chopped tomatoes. If using canned tomatoes, crush them by squeezing in your hand as you add to the pan.

4. Stir in red pepper flakes, olives, and capers. Simmer for 15 minutes.

5. Just before serving, toss in fresh basil and/or parsley.

Serve over GF pasta, polenta, or fish.

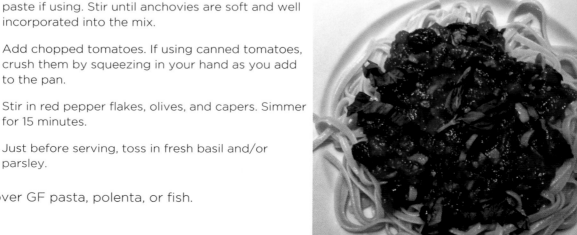

CRANBERRY SAUCE

(GF, SF, DF, NF, VG)

Prep time: 10 minutes

Cook time: 0

Serves: 6 as a Thanksgiving side; makes ~2 cups

Ingredients

1 bag (8–10 ounces) of fresh, raw cranberries

1 navel orange

1/8 cup maple sugar or honey (you can substitute coconut palm sugar)

1/4 teaspoon of ground cloves, optional (You can substitute ground ginger.)

Preparation

1. As you rinse the cranberries, sift through them with your hands to check for soft ones and discard any that you find.

2. Peel orange and remove as much pith as possible. There shouldn't be any seeds in a navel orange, but remove any if they are present.

3. Put all ingredients into a blender or Vitamix, and blend to desired consistency.

4. It's ready to serve. This recipe can also be made a day ahead of time and stored in the refrigerator.

Note: This is a great recipe to play around with the amount of sugar you add, gradually decreasing the amount. Play with it and see how low you can go. It will depend on the sweetness of the orange.

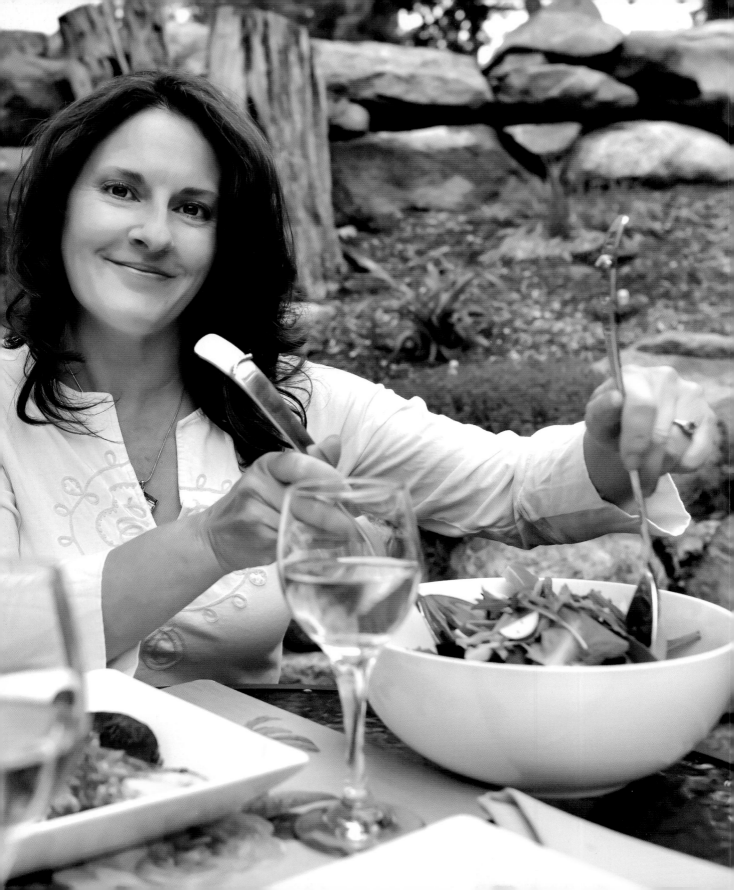

SALAD DRESSINGS

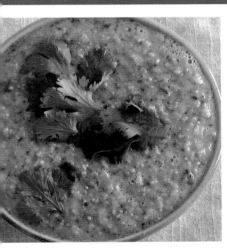 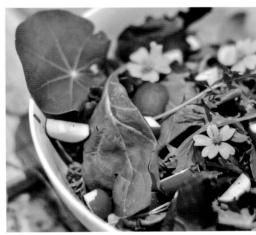 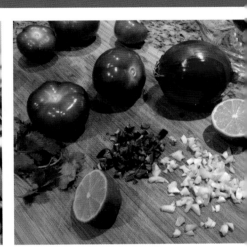

SNACKS

OLD-FASHIONED, IN FASHION, LEMON, AND OLIVE OIL

(GF, SF, DF, NF, VG, ED)

Ingredients

> Juice from 1/2–1 lemon
>
> EVOO in ~equal volume to the lemon
>
> Salt and pepper to taste

There is no preparation for this dressing other than to squeeze the lemon. Simply drizzle the EVOO over your salad, and then squeeze the lemon on top. You can use a net to catch the lemon seeds, or use a citrus reamer to extract the juice, and then pour it over the salad. Add S&P to taste, and mix well with salad tongs. There's a reason why this dressing remains a favorite in Italy and in my household. It's simply delicious.

MANGO-LIME DRESSING

(GF, SF, DF, NF, VG, ED)

Ingredients

> 1 medium mango
>
> 2 shallots
>
> Juice of 1 lime
>
> 1/2-inch piece of fresh ginger (can
>   substitute white or black pepper to taste)
>
> 1/2 cup EVOO

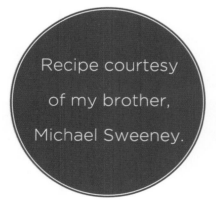

Recipe courtesy of my brother, Michael Sweeney.

Preparation

1. Chop shallots and ginger, and peel/pit mango.

2. Add mango to a food processor, blender, or Vitamix and purée.

3. Add lime juice, ginger, and shallots and mix well.

4. Slowly add EVOO until desired consistency is achieved.

Tip: Use on fruit salad, fish, and green salads.

ORANGE-GINGER DRESSING

(GF, SF, DF, NF, VG, ED)

Ingredients

- 4 tablespoons of freshly squeezed orange juice (juice from 1/2–1 orange)
- 4 tablespoons of EVOO
- 1 teaspoon finely chopped or grated fresh ginger
  (you can also use fresh ginger juice)
- 1 teaspoon fresh or dried oregano
- Salt and pepper to taste

Preparation

1. Squeeze juice from orange using a reamer. Pour into a bowl or bottle.

2. Mix remaining ingredients with orange juice. Shake or stir well. Use immediately. This dressing can be saved in the refrigerator for up to two days. It's best to make fresh when using freshly squeezed juice.

CREAMY GREENS DRESSING

(GF, SF, DF, NF, VG, ED)

Ingredients

- 1 cup parsley
- 1/2 avocado
- 2 cloves of garlic
- Juice of 1/2 a lemon
- 1/2 teaspoon salt
- 3 tablespoons water (to desired consistency)

Preparation

Put first five ingredients plus 1 TBSP of water in a Nutribullet, Vitamix, chopper, or blender. Blend until creamy, but do not overblend, as it may get too thick. Add more water as needed to attain desired consistency. A smaller vessel such as the Nutribullet or chopper works best because of the small volume, but any of these will do. If you are using a blender or Vitamix I recommend chopping the garlic first to ensure it doesn't remain one large piece.

SNACKS

Meals should typically be eaten every four hours, but see what your needs are. If you get very hungry two hours after a meal, you may want to tweak your macronutrient ratio to better suit your body's needs and sustain you longer. For example, if you notice that you get hungry within two hours every time you eat a meal made of predominantly carbohydrates, you should consider increasing the amount of protein next time and vice versa.

Having said that, there are still occasions when a snack is necessary between meals, especially if you are physically active. Be sure to eat a heavier snack at least an hour before a workout. A lighter snack can be eaten 30 minutes before a workout. Experiment with timing. Each individual and each workout is different.

Here are some healthy snack choices; eat only those which agree with your body, and be sure to rotate them just as you would a meal.

- **Nuts.** First, be sure nuts agree with you (you properly digest nuts) by observing your reaction immediately after eating and for the next two days. Some people react to nuts 1–2 days later, when the nuts reach the intestines.

- **Fresh fruit.** The earlier in the day you eat fruit, the better.

- **Dates or other dried fruit.** It's best not to overdo dried fruit, as it can be drying to the intestines. Also, be sure to buy organic with nothing added (Dried fruit often has sugar and/or flour added when bought in bulk. Be sure to read labels!)

- **Larabars; Kit bars; Pure bars; Raw crunch bars.** I only recommend processed foods such as these in a pinch or for pre- and post-workouts. As far as bars go, these are simple and organic.

- **Hummus and veggies**. Alone or spread in a coconut wrap. Observe your reaction to hummus as recommended for nuts.

- **Salsa and veggies**. (See recipe on page 157.)

- **Guacamole and veggies (in coconut wrap).** (See guacamole recipe on page 156.)

- **Avocado**. Place slices in a coconut wrap (see resources) or just slice it open, drizzle with EVOO, S&P if desired, and scoop with spoon.

- **Yogurt.** Only if it does not contain added sugar or anything other than milk and cultures. Yogurt is one of the most ruined snack items on the store shelf because of all of the added sugar and preservatives. Also, yogurt with fruit added is not recommended because the fruit is often bruised, overripe, underripe, or rejected for sale for some other reason so they dump it in your yogurt! Buy organic, but remember that just because the yogurt comes from a reputable organic brand doesn't mean it's good for you. Read the labels! I recommend plain, full-fat yogurt to which you can add your own honey or stevia to sweeten it if desired. Cacao nibs or vanilla also make a good addition.

- **Organic fresh cheese.** If dairy agrees with you, a quality cheese, preferably raw, makes a substantial snack. This is a snack that should be eaten sparingly.

- **Sardines.** These don't always travel well, but they're handy for a quick snack at home. (See recipe on page 154.)

- **Coconut pieces (no preservatives added) or a fresh young coconut.**

- **Homemade scones.** (See recipe on page 176.)

- **Homemade granola.** (See recipe on page 158.)

- **Leftovers.** The best snack you can have between lunch and dinner is some of your leftover lunch. What I often do is save a small amount of my lunch and eat it around 4–4:30 as a snack if I'm planning to work out in the evening.

SARDINES

(GF, SF, DF, NF, ED)

Prep time: 5 minutes

Cook time: 0

Serves 2

Ingredients

    1 can of sardines (~3.75 oz.) packed in spring water,
      preferably with bones for calcium

    Your choice of: juice from 1/2 lemon or 1 tablespoon of mustard
      mixed with 1 tablespoon EVOO

    Your favorite salad greens

Preparation

1. Open the can of sardines and put on a plate.

2. Squeeze lemon on top of sardines and eat, or

3. Mix mustard and EVOO or use mustard dressing and drizzle on top of sardines.

4. Place sardines atop a bed of greens for a well-rounded snack or lunch.

ENDIVE WITH BLUE CHEESE

(GF, SF, NF, VG)

Prep time: 5–10 minutes

Cook time: 0

Serves 2

Ingredients

1–2 heads of endive, depending on size

6 ounces of fresh blue cheese, preferably organic and raw

EVOO

Preparation

1. Peel and wash endive leaves. Dry leaves with salad spinner and/or paper towel.

2. Cut blue cheese into small chucks or cubes, like crumbles.

3. Drizzle with small amount of EVOO.

GUACAMOLE

(GF, SF, DF, NF, VG, ED)

Prep time: 15 minutes

Cook time: 0

Serves 2–4

Ingredients

2 avocados

2 lemons, juiced (limes work as well)

2-plus cloves of garlic, peeled
   (or use 1/2 red onion, but I don't recommend both garlic and onion)

1/2–1 bunch of cilantro

1/2 jalapeño or other hot pepper (optional)
   (You can substitute 1/2 tsp. red pepper flakes if desired.)

2 tablespoon EVOO

Salt and pepper to taste

Preparation

1. Place half of each ingredient in a chopper or blender. Blend until mixed but not smooth.

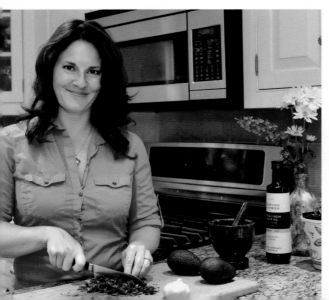

2. Taste and decide how much more of each of the other ingredients to add along with your second avocado (so it is to your liking).

3. Add remaining ingredients and blend. I prefer my guacamole a bit chunky, but blend until your desired texture is reached. If you don't have a chopper or blender or you like it really chunky, you can mix ingredients in a bowl, stirring and crushing the avocado with a spoon or use a mortar and pestle. Serve with your favorite dipping food (veggie or healthy chip) or eat alone for an even easier snack. Guacamole also tastes great over a mild white fish.

SALSA VERDE

(GF, SF, DF, NF, VG, ED)

Prep time: 15 minutes

Cook time: 0

Serves 6

Ingredients

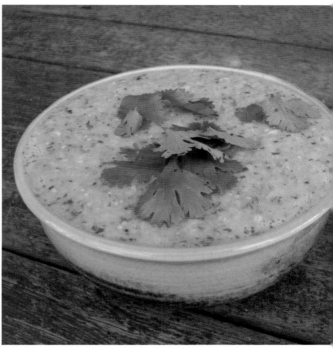

2 quarts water

1 pound tomatillos

3 large garlic cloves

1/2 chopped onion

1 tablespoon EVOO

1/4 cup lime juice
   (~2 limes. You can also use lemons.)

1/2 cup cilantro

1/2–1 jalapeño pepper

1/2 teaspoon salt

Black pepper to taste

Preparation

1. Get water boiling in a large pot. Husk tomatillos and chop onion, garlic, and pepper.

2. Once water is boiling, add tomatillos and boil for three minutes. Meanwhile, juice the limes.

3. After three minutes, drain the tomatillos and add them to a blender, food processor, or Vitamix.

4. Add in remaining ingredients and blend for a few seconds. Do not overblend.

5. Store salsa in a sealed container in the refrigerator up to four to seven days.

Serving Suggestion: Eat as a snack with veggies or chips. Serve as a sauce over a mild white fish.

AROMATIC GRANOLA

(GF, SF, DF, VG)

Prep time: 5–10 minutes

Cook time: 45 minutes

Serves 4

If you feel the need for something sweet, try this granola. The spices are so delicious, and they quench my need for a sweet.

Ingredients

2 cups GF rolled oats

1/3–1/2 cup chopped raw walnuts (Omit if you can't digest nuts.)

1/4 cup raw pumpkin seeds

1/4 cup hemp seeds (You can also use sesame seeds or sunflower seeds.)

1 tablespoon cinnamon

1 teaspoon ground cloves

1 teaspoon nutmeg

1 teaspoon cardamom

1/2 teaspoon ground ginger (can substitute 1-1/2 tablespoons chopped candied ginger pieces)

1/4 cup unsweetened shredded coconut (optional)

1/2 teaspoon salt

2 tablespoons coconut oil, melted

1/4 cup maple syrup

1–2 teaspoons honey (optional)

Preparation

1. Preheat oven to 300°F.

2. Add all ingredients except the honey to a large bowl in the order listed. Mix well.

3. Pour into a 13 x 9 glass baking dish (or a cookie sheet lined with parchment paper) spreading into one layer. Bake 45 minutes, stirring once halfway through cooking time.

4. Once you take it out of the oven, test the sweetness. If you like it sweeter, stir in the honey 1 tsp. at a time.

Note: Baking on low heat maintains nutrients. If you're pressed for time, you can bake at 325°F for 30 minutes. If you've got plenty of time, try 250°F for one hour.

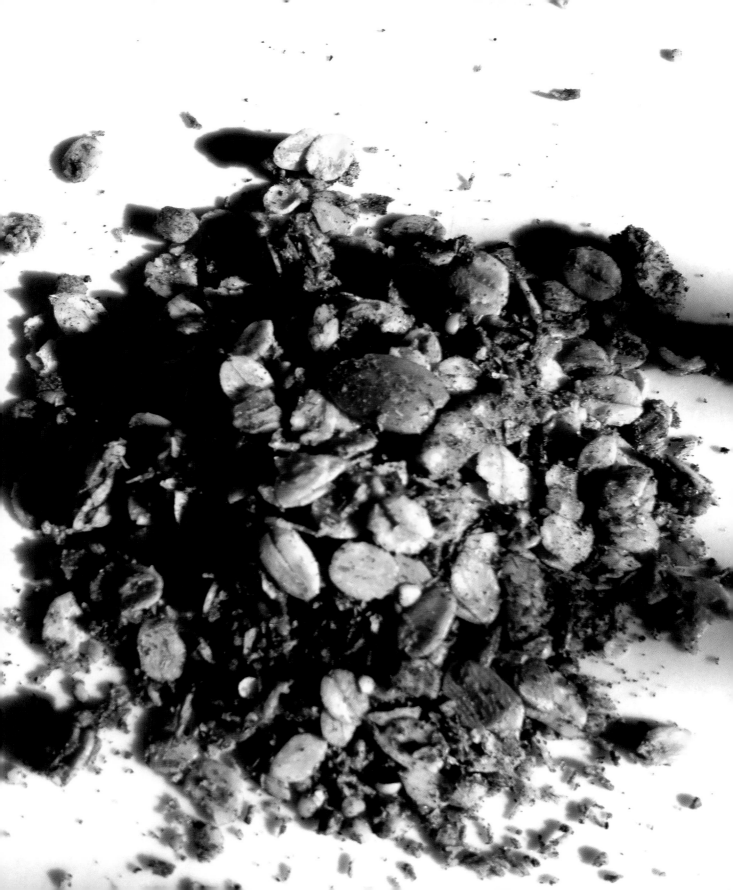

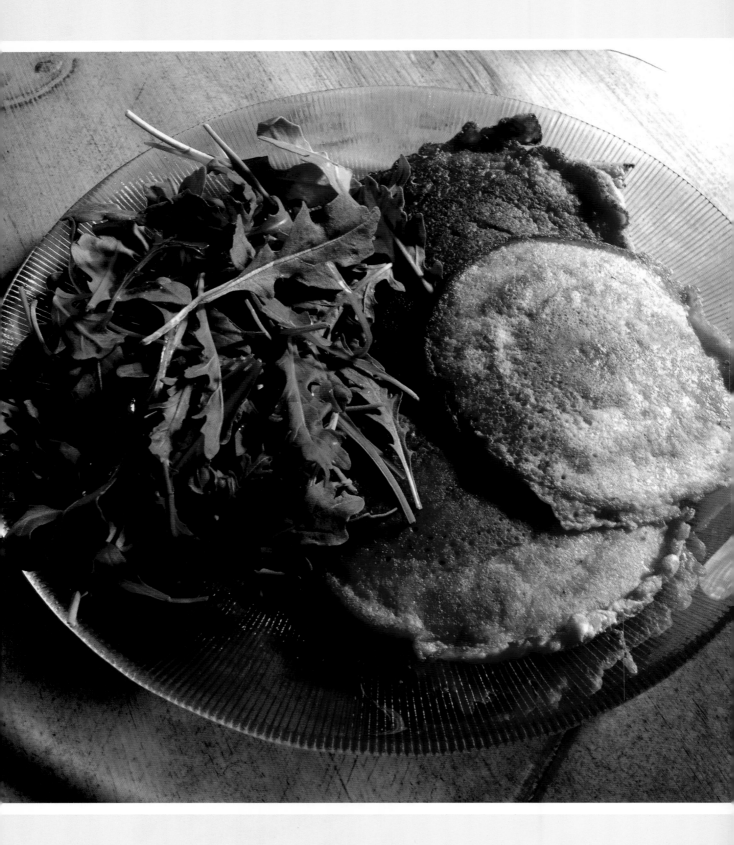

BREAKFAST

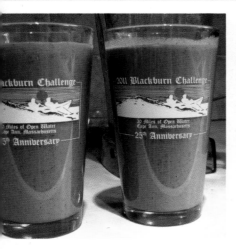
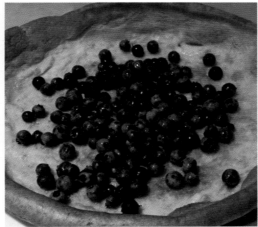
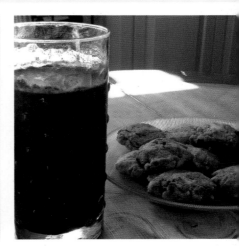

ALMOND MILK

(GF, SF, DF, VG)

Prep time: 5 minutes, plus 8–16 hours hands-off

Cook time: 0

Serves 2

Ingredients

3/4 cup raw, organic almonds (I prefer skinless, but it's up to you.)

2 cups water, plus extra for soaking

Preparation

1. Put almonds in a glass bowl and cover them completely with water. Soak overnight.

2. Drain almonds and blend in blender, Nutribullet, or Vitamix with 1 cup of water. Add remaining 1 cup of water and blend on high speed until smooth.

3. I use the almond milk as is, but you can strain it if needed (some blenders leave larger chunks than others). Use a sieve or cheesecloth to strain if desired.

Tips: Refrigerate and use nut milks within two days of making.

Once you've soaked nuts, you must either use them right away or dry them so they don't mold. To dry, place nuts in one layer on an oven-proof tray and slow roast at 110°F until crunchy (not rubbery). This takes 24–36 hours.

Mix almond milk in a blender or Vitamix with 1/4 cup almonds, 2 tablespoons almond butter, and 1/2 a banana (or 2 TBSP squash/pumpkin purée) for a delicious smoothie.

CASHEW MILK

(GF, SF, DF, VG)

Prep time: 5 minutes, plus 30 minutes hands-off

Cook time: 0

Serves 2-4

Ingredients

1 cup raw, organic cashews

3 cups water, plus additional for soaking

1/2 teaspoon vanilla, optional

10-15 cardamom seeds (seeds, not whole pods, optional)

Preparation

1. Add cashews to a glass bowl, and add enough water to cover them. Soak 30 minutes.

2. Drain and then add soaked cashews, cardamom, and 3 cups of fresh water to a blender, Nutribullet, or Vitamix. Blend on high speed until smooth.

3. Once blended, I recommend tasting it before adding vanilla. I sometimes make oatmeal with the cashew milk, and if there is any remaining, I add a touch of vanilla and drink it.

Notes:

If you have a Nutribullet or Vitamix, the milk should be smooth enough to drink or use as is. If not, use cheesecloth or a sieve to strain it.

Cashews, like peanuts, are more susceptible to mold than most nuts and should not be soaked for long periods of time (such as overnight). Once soaked, cashews should be eaten within a few hours.

HEMP MILK

(GF, SF, DF, NF, VG, ED)

Prep time: 5 minutes

Cook time: 0

Serves 1

Ingredients

1/4 cup hemp hearts (see resources)

1 cup water

1/2 teaspoon vanilla (optional)

Preparation

Add all ingredients to a Vitamix, Nutribullet, or high-speed blender and blend on high for about 30 seconds or until smooth. Drink up or use in your favorite breakfast recipe.

COCONUT BERRY SMOOTHIE

(GF, SF, DF, VG)

Prep time: 10 minutes

Cook time: 0

Serves 2

Ingredients

> 22.4 ounces (660 ml) coconut water
>
> 2 fresh dates
>
> 1/2 a banana
>
> 2 tablespoons coconut manna (coconut butter or meat)
>
> 1 tablespoon protein powder (I use Navitas Naturals superfood blend.)
>
> 2 tablespoons shredded coconut (unsweetened)
>
> 1/4 cup frozen blueberries (can substitute your favorite berry)

Preparation

Add all ingredients to a blender or Vitamix. Blend until smooth or desired consistency.

Note: Coconut manna (a.k.a. coconut butter) and Navitas Naturals superfood blend can be found at most grocery stores, including Whole Foods. See my resources section for more information.

A note on smoothies and juices: Go easy on the fruit (because of the added sugar), and add some type of fat (EVOO, coconut oil, or avocado) to help absorb the nutrients.

Serving Suggestion: Serve with scones.

CASHEW SMOOTHIE

(GF, SF, DF, VG)

Prep time: 10 minutes

Cook time: 0

Serves 2

Ingredients

    22.4 ounces (660 ml) coconut water

    1/2 banana (Use whole banana for thicker consistency.)

    2 tablespoons cashew butter

    1/4 cup cashews

    2 tablespoons coconut manna (coconut butter or meat)

    2 tablespoons flax seeds (optional)

    2 tablespoons shredded coconut, unsweetened (optional)

    1/4 teaspoon vanilla (optional)

Preparation

Add all ingredients to a blender or Vitamix. Blend until smooth or desired consistency is reached.

Note: Coconut manna (a.k.a. coconut butter) can be found at most grocery stores, including Whole Foods.

COCONUT ALMOND SMOOTHIE

(GF, SF, DF, VG)

Prep time: 10 minutes

Cook time: 0

Serves 2

Ingredients

22.4 ounces (660 ml) coconut water

1/2-1 banana, depending on how thick you want it
   (can substitute 2 TBSP pumpkin purée)

2 tablespoons almond butter

1/4 cup raw almonds

2 tablespoons coconut manna (coconut butter or meat)

2 fresh dates, pitted

2 tablespoons shredded coconut, unsweetened

Preparation

Add all ingredients to a blender or Vitamix. Blend until smooth or desired consistency is reached. Add second half of banana if consistency is too thin for your liking.

Note: Coconut manna (a.k.a. coconut butter) can be found at most grocery stores, including Whole Foods.

In the beginning, I wasn't diggin' the green smoothie movement. My husband would concoct various forms of the green smoothie, and I would take one sip and run for the hills. Then one day he hit a home run with this recipe. Sometimes I eat it with a spoon so it feels like I'm eating a salad. In fact, I am eating a salad, and that's why it tastes so good.

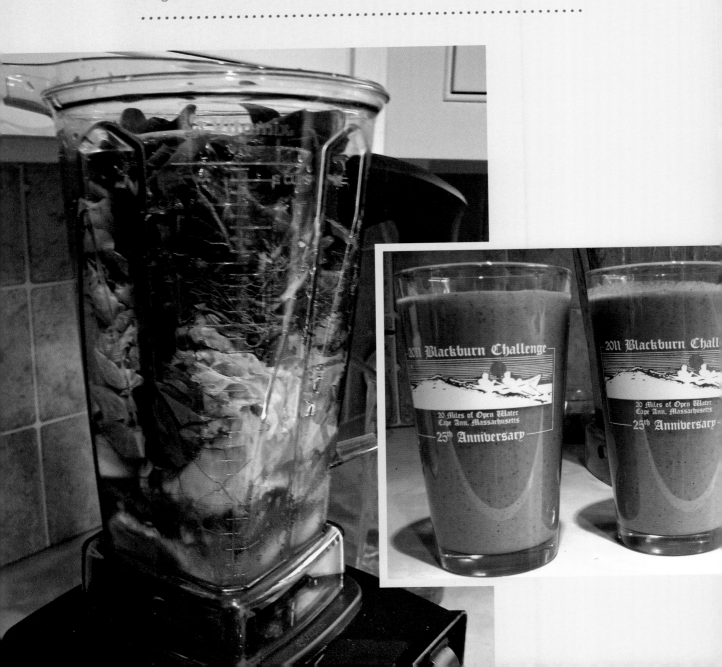

INFAMOUS GREEN SMOOTHIE

(GF, SF, DF, NF, VG, ED)

Prep time: 10 minutes

Cooking time: 0

Serves 2

Ingredients

- 1 cup of water, more or less depending on desired thickness
- 1 apple, cored and roughly chopped (I like to use a gala or pink lady. You can also use a pear.)
- 1/2 lemon (with rind if it's organic and you have a Vitamix or other heavy-duty blade)
- 6-inch piece of fennel, along with a pinch of fennel greens (can substitute with celery)
- 3 ounces of any greens or 1/2 head of lettuce (I like romaine, red leaf lettuce, or arugula)
- 1 large handful of parsley (can include stems)
- 1 large handful of cilantro (can include stems)
- 1 teaspoon turmeric powder (or 1/4-inch piece of turmeric root, optional)
- 1 teaspoon ginger powder (or 1/2-inch piece of ginger root, optional)
- 2 tablespoons EVOO
- 1 teaspoon sea salt
- 1/2 teaspoon cayenne pepper or black pepper

Preparation

1. Add water to Vitamix. Add remaining ingredients in the order listed and mix until blended.

2. If you have a Vitamix, you can get away with roughly chopping the apple and lemon, but if you have a blender, you may need to chop into smaller pieces.

Note: If you have beet greens that you don't know what to do with, throw some in this smoothie. I don't recommend more than 3-5 leaves.

SAVORY OMELET

(GF, SF, DF, NF, VG)

Prep time: 10 minutes

Cook time: 5–10 minutes

Serves 1

Ingredients

3 eggs (or however many you'd like)

1 cup of your favorite leafy green (chard, spinach, arugula, or a combo)

1/2 bell or poblano pepper

5 sage leaves (can also use basil, oregano, or your favorite herb, preferably fresh, but dried is okay)

2 radishes (optional)

Salt and pepper to taste

Preparation

1. Roughly chop radishes, greens, pepper, and herbs if using fresh.

2. Gently mix eggs in a bowl, mix in S&P and then remaining ingredients.

3. Heat butter or EVOO over low-medium heat and add omelet mixture. Cook about three to five minutes, according to how brown you like it, and then flip and cook about three to five minutes.

MEHUL'S NUTTY PANCAKES

(GF, SF, DF, VG)

Prep time: 5 minutes

Cook time: 15 minutes

Makes 10–12 pancakes

Ingredients

> 1 large egg
>
> 1-1/4 cup coconut water
>
> 1 tablespoon coconut oil, melted preferred (plus extra for cooking)
>
> 1/4 cup coconut flour, sifted if desired
>
> 1/4 cup garbanzo bean flour
>
> 1/2 cup chestnut flour
>
> 1 teaspoon baking soda
>
> 1 scoop (or pinch) of stevia*
>
> 1/4 cup shredded coconut, unsweetened

Preparation

1. Mix dry ingredients in a large bowl.

2. Mix wet ingredients in a small bowl.

3. Add wet ingredients to dry ingredients and mix well.

4. Heat frying pan over medium-low heat and add coconut oil.

5. Add 1/4 cup of batter to the pan for each pancake. Cook ~two minutes each side, or flip when bubbles appear on top of pancake.

6. Serve as is or with maple syrup, melted coconut oil, or nut butter.

*This refers to the tiny scoop that comes with many bottles of pure powdered stevia and can be approximated by a pinch if you don't have a scoop. Generally, 1 teaspoon of sugar = 1 pinch of pure powdered stevia = 2–4 drops liquid concentrate stevia.

ALMOND PANCAKES

(GF, SF, DF, VG)

Prep time: 5 minutes

Cook time: 15 minutes

Serves 4

Ingredients

    1 large egg

    1-1/3 cup almond milk

    1 tablespoon coconut oil

    1/2 cup chestnut flour*

    1/4 cup almond meal (or flour)

    1/4 cup coconut flour

    1 teaspoon baking soda

    1 scoop (pinch) stevia**

    3 tablespoon crushed almonds

    Dash of almond extract (optional)

* If you don't have chestnut flour, you can use 1/2 cup coconut flour and 1/2 cup almond meal (or flour). In this case I recommend the alternate preparation. **This refers to the tiny scoop that comes with many bottles of pure powdered stevia and can be approximated by a pinch if you don't have a scoop. Generally, 1 teaspoon of sugar = 1 pinch of pure powdered stevia = 2-4 drops liquid concentrate stevia.

Preparation

1. Mix dry ingredients in a large bowl.

2. Mix wet ingredients in a small bowl.

3. Add wet ingredients to dry ingredients, and mix well.

4. Heat frying pan over medium heat, and add coconut oil.

5. Add 1/4 cup batter to the pan for each pancake. Flip when bubbles appear.

6. Top with coconut oil, and serve as is or with maple syrup.

Alternate preparation: If you don't feel like standing over the stove flipping pancakes, you can bake them instead. Form pancakes about 1/4-inch thick, and place on parchment paper or cookie sheet. Bake at 365°F for ten minutes.

PUMPKIN PANCAKES

(GF, SF, DF, NF, VG)

Prep time: 5 minutes

Cook time: 15 minutes

Serves 2–4

Ingredients

  3 large eggs (or 4 smaller eggs)

  2/3 cup of pumpkin purée (packed)

  1 teaspoon vanilla extract

  3 tablespoons cinnamon

  Ground ginger to taste (~1 teaspoon)

  Ground nutmeg to taste (~1 teaspoon)

  Ground cloves to taste (~1/2 teaspoon)

  Ground cardamom to taste (~1/2 teaspoon)

  Your favorite oil for cooking (I use butter or coconut oil. DF and NF eaters should choose accordingly.)

Preparation

1. Crack eggs in a bowl, and mix with a fork. Add all remaining ingredients and mix well. Alternatively, You can add all ingredients to a blender or Vitamix to mix if you wish. Do not over mix or pancakes may not flip as easily.

2. Add butter or coconut oil to a frying pan over medium to medium-low heat. Cook as you would any pancake (use 1/4–1/3 cup of batter for each pancake), flipping halfway through cooking.

3. Eat alone or with maple syrup, apple cider syrup, or honey.

Note: The first time you try these you may find they need sweetness. Eventually, you may enjoy them without syrup or added sweetness.

ALL-DAY CARROT PANCAKES

(GF, SF, DF, NF, VG)

Prep time: 5 minutes

Cook time: 10 minutes

Serves 2

Adapted from
*The Whole-Food Guide
to Overcoming Irritable
Bowel Syndrome*
by Laura J. Knoff, NC
I find these pancakes
delightfully sweet,
yet perfect any
time of day.

Ingredients

1 large raw carrot or 1 cup of cooked carrots
(see note)

4 eggs

3 tablespoons EVOO

1/2–1 teaspoon cinnamon

Preparation

1. In a blender, add the eggs, carrot, cinnamon, and 1 TBSP of EVOO. Blend until smooth.

2. Heat the remaining EVOO in a frying pan over medium heat. When hot, add pancake batter. Cook as you would any pancake (these take a little longer on the first side).

Notes: This recipe is great if you have leftover cooked carrots (plain). You can also steam carrots to use for this recipe or use a raw carrot if you have a blender with a sharp enough blade to chop them until smooth (a Vitamix works well).

Tips: The sweeter the carrot, the sweeter the pancake. I recommend buying carrots from a local farm, as they tend to be sweeter. I eat these pancakes on their own, but you can top with apple cider syrup, apple sauce, almond butter (won't be nut-free), or anything you choose. I was a bit skeptical of this recipe at first, but I fell in love at first bite.

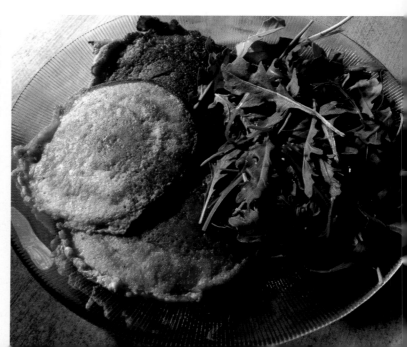

BREAKFAST POPOVER

(GF, SF, NF, VG)

Prep time: 5 minutes

Cook time: 12 minutes

Makes 1 popover in a 9-inch pie plate. I can eat a whole one, but many people eat half. 1 popover serves 1–2, depending on your appetite!

Ingredients

> 1/2 cup chestnut flour (or gluten-free oat flour)
>
> 1/2 cup milk
>
> 2 eggs
>
> 1-1/2 tablespoon butter

Preparation

1. Preheat oven to 475°F.

2. Beat eggs with a fork, and then add milk and flour. Mix well, but do not overmix—there may be a few small lumps.

3. Put butter in a 9" pie plate and place in the oven one to two minutes to melt butter. Remove pie plate from oven once butter is melted.

4. Pour batter into pie plate on top of melted butter and place in oven for 12–14 minutes or until just beginning to brown on the edges.
   Top with fresh or frozen berries, honey, butter, lemon juice, or lemon curd.

If you prefer to avoid milk, you can substitute almond milk (it will not be nut-free) or hemp milk. The recipe will still contain butter so it will not be completely dairy-free, but many dairy-free people can tolerate butter.

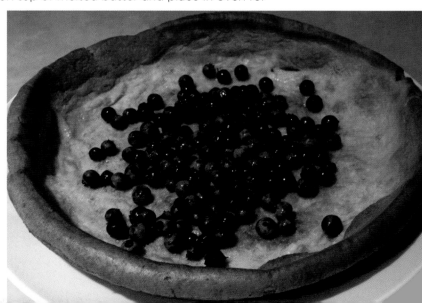

SCONES

(GF, SF, DF, VG)

Prep time: 10 minutes

Cook time: 12 minutes

Makes 8 scones

Ingredients

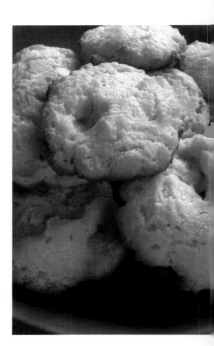

    6 eggs

    1/2 cup coconut flour

    1/4 cup coconut oil, melted if possible

    3/4 teaspoon baking soda

    2 scoops* stevia or 1 teaspoon coconut palm sugar

    Dash of salt

    1 teaspoon vanilla

    2 tablespoons currants (optional)

    2 tablespoons Superfood Blend (protein smoothie mix)
      by Navitas Naturals (optional)

Preparation

1. Preheat oven to 375°F. Place coconut oil in an oven-proof bowl (I use Pyrex.) and place in oven to melt (one to two minutes). Don't worry if it is not exactly 1/4 cup.

2. Whisk eggs in a bowl. Add all other ingredients and mix well. Use your hands to mix if necessary. Don't worry if some lumps of coconut oil remain.

3. Form batter into cookie-size aliquots about 1/2 inch thick, and place on parchment paper, cookie sheet, or silicone pad (if you use parchment paper or silicone pad it's best to place them on a cookie sheet because the coconut oil can run).

4. Place scones in the oven and bake for 12 minutes or until just barely browning on the edges. Do not overcook, as they could become dry. Eat as is, drizzle with honey, or top with berries or jam. Bionaturae makes delicious fruit spreads that go well with these scones. Enjoy!

*This refers to the tiny scoop that comes with many bottles of pure powdered stevia and can be approximated by a pinch if you don't have a scoop. Generally, 1 teaspoon of sugar = 1 pinch of pure powdered stevia = 2–4 drops liquid concentrate stevia.

DESSERTS

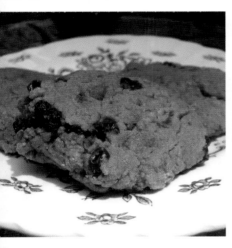
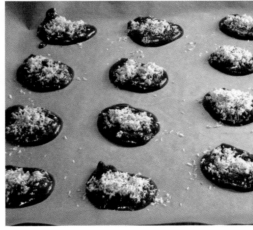
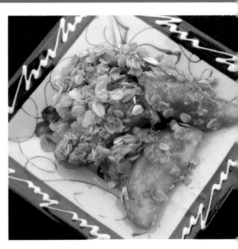

CHESTNUT COOKIES

(GF, SF, VG)

Prep time: 15 minutes

Cook time: 12 minutes

Makes 12 cookies

Ingredients

1/3 cup (6 TBSP) unsalted butter, room temperature

1 egg, preferably room temperature

1/2 cup chestnut purée, fairly packed (see resources)

1-1/4 cup chestnut flour

1 teaspoon vanilla

1/8 cup coconut palm sugar (can substitute 1 scoop* stevia)

1 level teaspoon baking soda

1/2 cup chocolate chips, optional

Preparation

1. Preheat oven to 350°F.

2. Mix butter, egg, and vanilla with electric beater on medium-low. Add in chestnut purée and continue to mix. Note: If you find it difficult to measure the purée exactly, it's better to use too much than too little. Similarly, if you have just over 1/2 cup of purée remaining from the last batch you made, feel free to use it all.

3. Add chestnut flour, sugar, and baking soda and continue to mix on medium-low until blended. If it's crumbly, you can finish mixing with your hands, but do not overmix.

4. Form batter into balls ~1 tablespoon in size and flatten slightly. Place on parchment paper lined cookie sheet and bake for 10–12 minutes.

   Alternatives to chocolate chips: Instead of chocolate chips, try adding currants, walnuts, shredded coconut, or cacao nibs. These cookies are also delicious drizzled with dark chocolate. I melt my favorite dark chocolate (such as Taza 87 percent dark) in a Pyrex bowl over gently boiling water and drizzle it on top of cooled cookies. See dark chocolate delights recipe for more info on melting chocolate in a makeshift double boiler.

Notes:

For dairy-free cookies, substitute melted coconut oil for the butter. Cookies will be thinner.

I've made this recipe using only 1 cup of chestnut flour, and it works well. The cookies are moist-er but a little crumbly. 1 cup of flour will do, but if you don't want to risk your cookie crumbling, use an additional 1/4 cup.

I often leave out the sweetener when making these cookies. I find the chestnut and vanilla sweet enough. This may be a good recipe for slowly weaning yourself off sugar/added sweetener.

This recipe can be made without the chestnut purée, but it's more delicious and moist with it. Choose purée that is 100 percent chestnuts (no sugar or anything else added). See resources for brands and stores.

When doubling this recipe, I've found the ratios to be different. I double the butter, egg, and sugar but add only 1-1/2 cups of flour, 1-1/2 tsp. of vanilla, and 1-1/2 tsp. baking soda.

*This refers to the tiny scoop that comes with many bottles of pure powdered stevia and can be approximated by a pinch if you don't have a scoop. Generally, 1 teaspoon of sugar = 1 pinch of pure powdered stevia = 2–4 drops liquid concentrate stevia.

• •

While visiting Portugal in November 2013, I was pleasantly surprised to arrive in peak chestnut season. The sweet smell of roasted chestnuts rose up from nearly every street corner. I found myself asking, more than once, "Are we due for another bag of chestnuts? It's been almost 15 minutes." The chestnuts were soft, warm, and sweeter than I imagined. Divine! When I came home, I was in a chestnut state of mind. These cookies were born from my wonderful Portugal experience and a desire to continue enjoying these perfect nuts.

• •

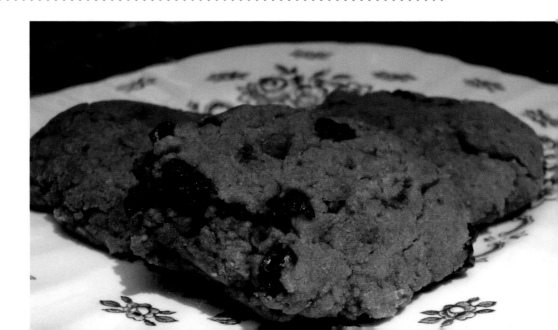

ALMOND CAKE

(GF, SF, DF*, VG)

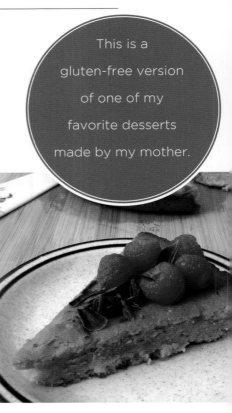

This is a gluten-free version of one of my favorite desserts made by my mother.

Prep time: 15–20 minutes

Cook time: 30 minutes

Ingredients

- 10 ounces gluten-free almond paste (see resources)
- 1/2 cup almond flour
- 2 tablespoons coconut palm sugar
- 1 stick (8 TBSP) of unsalted butter at room temperature, plus a little extra for greasing
- 3 eggs at room temperature

Preparation

1. Take butter and eggs out of refrigerator and bring to room temperature at least 30 minutes before getting started. Preheat oven to 350°F.

2. Grease a small 8" cake or tart pan with butter.

3. Cut almond paste into small pieces (a butter knife works well), or grate it using a cheese grater or potato peeler.

4. Add paste to a large mixing bowl with butter (one stick) and sugar. Mix with an electric mixer on low speed until blended.

5. Add eggs one at a time and continue mixing on low as you add them. Then mix on high speed until batter is light and fluffy, about two to three minutes.

6. Fold the almond flour into the batter with a spatula.

7. Spread batter into greased pan, and bake for 30 minutes or until just golden.

. . . .

Serving Suggestion: This cake is delicious as is, topped with fresh raspberries, dusted with cocoa powder, or drizzled with dark chocolate (see dark chocolate delights for information on melting chocolate to use for your drizzle).

. . . .

Note: You can make your own almond flour by adding 1/3 cup of raw skinless almonds (I use Marcona almonds.) to a Vitamix and blending on high for 8–10 seconds. Do not overblend, as it will become pasty and be difficult to remove from the Vitamix.

*This recipe may be ok for you if you tolerate butter.

APPLE CRISP

(GF, SF, DF*, NF, VG)

Prep time: 15–20 minutes

Cook time: 30–35 minutes

Serves: 6

Ingredients

5 cups of apples (about 5 apples. You can also use pears, peaches, or berries)

3/4 cup rolled oats, gluten free

1/4 cup maple sugar

(can substitute coconut palm sugar)

1/4 cup (4 TBSP) butter

1/4 teaspoon cinnamon

1/4 teaspoon nutmeg

1/4 teaspoon ground ginger

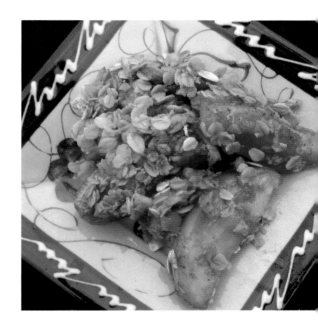

Preparation

1. Preheat oven to 375°F.

2. Wash and evenly slice apples (using an apple slicer helps if you have one). I don't peel the apples, but you can if you prefer.

3. Place sliced apples in an 8 x 8 x 2 oven-proof baking dish or 8-9-inch pie plate. Stir in maple sugar.

4. In a separate bowl, mix oats and spices. Using a butter knife, cut in the butter about a TBSP at a time (add 1 TBSP of butter at a time to the bowl and cut it into pieces with a butter knife allowing it to blend with oat mixture). Add butter in this way until the mixture looks like coarse crumbs. Do not overmix or melt the butter. Don't worry about it being 100 percent mixed.

5. Pour the oat mixture on top of the fruit. Bake for 30–35 minutes or until fruit is soft and topping is golden brown. Serve warm.

Note: The only dairy in this recipe is the butter, so it may be okay for those who are dairy-free but can tolerate butter.

*This recipe may be ok for you if you tolerate butter.

TAPIOCA

(GF, SF, DF, VG)

Prep time: 5 minutes

Cook time: 35–40 minutes

Serves: 4

Ingredients

3-1/2 cups water

6 tablespoons of tapioca, small pearl

13-1/2 ounce can (1-2/3 cup) of coconut milk (full fat)

2–3 tablespoons of coconut palm sugar or 2 scoops* of stevia, optional

1 teaspoon vanilla

1/4 teaspoon salt

2/3 cup of shredded coconut, unsweetened, optional

Preparation

1. Bring 3-1/2 cups of water to a boil. Add tapioca and cook with lid off over low-medium heat until opaque, about 17–20 minutes. Stir occasionally to prevent sticking.

2. While the tapioca is cooking, mix coconut milk in a bowl with sugar, vanilla, and salt.

3. After the tapioca has cooked and looks opaque and gelatinous, stir in the coconut milk mixture. Cook over low-medium heat for seven to eight minutes, stirring occasionally.

4. Stir in shredded coconut if desired, and cook an additional two minutes.

5. Pour tapioca into four heat-resistant bowls (like Pyrex or CorningWare), cover tightly with plastic wrap, and refrigerate for several hours. Serve cold as a pudding.

Note: I sometimes omit or limit the sugar and eat the tapioca right after it comes off the stove as a complement to my breakfast.

This recipe can be made nut-free by substituting milk for coconut milk (not dairy-free).

*This refers to the tiny scoop that comes with many bottles of pure powdered stevia and can be approximated by a pinch if you don't have a scoop. Generally, 1 teaspoon of sugar = 1 pinch of pure powdered stevia = 2-4 drops liquid concentrate stevia.

WARM CHOCOLATE CAKES

(GF, SF, NF, VG)

Prep time: 40 minutes

Cook time: 10–15 minutes

Makes 4–6 cakes

Ingredients

- 1/2 cup (1 stick) of unsalted butter
- 6–8 ounces dark chocolate (the better the quality, the better the final taste)
- 3 eggs, at room temperature
- 2 tablespoons of maple or palm sugar
- 1 teaspoon pure vanilla extract

Preparation

1. Preheat the oven to 400°F, and grease ovenproof bowls with butter. You can use four 6–8 ounce bowls or six 4–5 ounce bowls.

2. Cut butter and chocolate into pieces and place in a heat-proof bowl such as a Pyrex bowl. It helps to cut the chocolate smaller than the butter for equal melting time. Place bowl over a pot of simmering water and stir until melted. Remove from heat and let cool.

3. Separate eggs. Set whites aside and add yolks to a mixing bowl with 1 TBSP sugar. Using an electric mixer, mix on high until thick (slightly thinner than real whipped cream) and pale, about three minutes. Add vanilla and mix in gently.

4. Pour the cooled, melted chocolate-butter mixture into the whipped egg yolk mixture and fold in or mix gently until well blended.

5. In a separate bowl, beat the egg whites plus 1 TBSP sugar on medium speed until glossy and soft peaks form. Overbeating can cause the cakes to be flat.

6. Fold half the egg white mixture into the chocolate mixture, being careful not to overmix. Once incorporated, fold in the remaining half of the egg white mixture until well mixed.

7. Divide batter equally into your greased bowls and bake for 10–15 minutes depending on the consistency you desire. If you like a soft center, bake

for ten minutes (this is my preferred cooking time). If you prefer a more cake-like texture, cook for 12–15 minutes. Serve immediately.

Tip: You can make and distribute the batter several hours ahead of time, cover with plastic wrap, and refrigerate until you're ready to bake them. Take them out of the refrigerator about 30 minutes before you bake them and bake for an additional minute or two if they are still cool when you put them in the oven. If you don't finish them all (I can't imagine), you can cover and refrigerate them. The next day just take them out of the refrigerator 30–60 minutes before you want to eat them.

Note: The only dairy in these is the butter, so they may be okay for those who are dairy-free but can tolerate butter.

COCONUT-CAROB CANDIES

(GF, SF, DF, VG)

Prep time: 10–15 minutes

Chill time: 30–60 minutes

Adapted from
*The Whole-Food Guide
to Overcoming Irritable
Bowel Syndrome*
by Laura J. Knoff, NC
Carob is a great substitute
for chocolate
if you need one.

Ingredients

1 cup of coconut oil, melted

1/2 cup roasted carob powder*

(You can buy it roasted.)

*Carob is naturally sweet and alkalizing and does not contain caffeine or oxalic acid. As with chocolate, eat carob in moderation but feel guiltless when you do.

Preparation

1. Measure out the coconut oil and melt it in a saucepan if necessary. Once it's melted, double check that you have 1 cup.

2. Add the carob powder and mix until all lumps are removed. A whisk works well.

3. Pour the mixture into ice cube trays, filling each cube about 1/4–1/2 full.

4. Place tray in the freezer until the candy hardens. I usually leave it in the freezer at least one hour, but you can check it after 30 minutes. Once they've hardened you can pop them out of the tray as needed or pop them all out and store in a glass jar in the refrigerator or freezer.

Notes: These melt very quickly, so they cannot be left at room temperature (they'll turn liquid in warm temperature just like coconut oil). This also means they should not remain in your hand for long, but why would they?

I've made these by pouring the mix into a Pyrex pie plate instead of an ice tray. I chill it the same way, then pry the hardened mixture out of the plate onto a cutting board, and cut into bite-size pieces. If you choose this method, be careful with the glass when prying the hardened mixture out of the plate.

Tips: You can add chopped nuts or shredded coconut to the mixture before pouring it into the tray.

DARK CHOCOLATE DELIGHTS

(GF, SF, DF*, VG)

Prep time: 20–25 minutes

Cook time: 0 minutes

Cool time: 30 minutes

Makes 20 pieces

Ingredients

1 cup dark chocolate pieces *

2 tablespoons almond butter (I use sprouted almond butter.)

1 tablespoon maple syrup

1 teaspoon pure vanilla extract

2 tablespoon finely chopped pecans, toasted (optional)

1 teaspoon cinnamon

1 teaspoon ground cardamom

2 tablespoon unsweetened shredded coconut (toasted or raw) (optional)

* I use a different blend of chocolate each time I make this, whatever I have on hand, but always dark (55 percent will do, but 70 percent or more is best). My favorite blends usually include a small amount of dark chocolate flavored with cinnamon or chili pepper. If you are dairy-free, choose your chocolate accordingly.

Preparation

1. Melt the chocolate pieces in a double boiler if you have one. I don't own a double boiler, so I use a Pyrex bowl over a pot with simmering water. See picture.

2. Stir in the almond butter, maple syrup, and vanilla extract.

3. Stir in the pecans, cinnamon, and cardamom.

4. Line a tray with wax or parchment paper. Drop chocolate mixture onto tray using TBSP-sized portions approximately 1/2-inch thick (don't worry if the chocolate runs a bit and is thinner). The chocolate should "dollop" off the spoon in an egg shape.

5. Sprinkle each piece with coconut and refrigerate for 30 minutes or until firm.

6. Serve or store in an airtight container in the refrigerator.

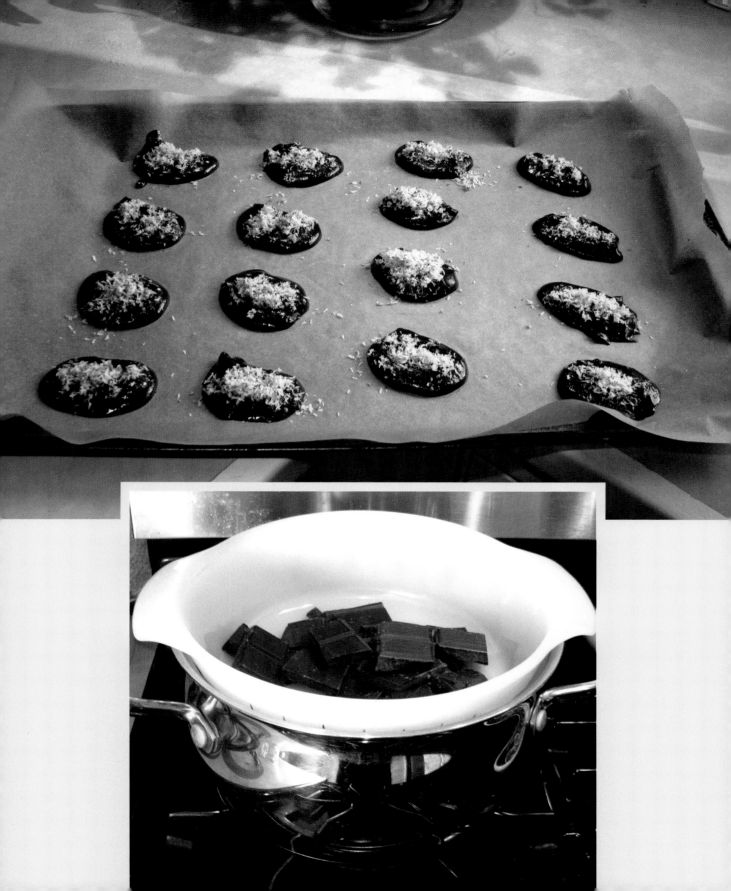

FUN FOOD AND KITCHEN TIPS

- Add a pinch of cardamom to your coffee to reduce acidity.

- Squeeze half a lemon into 6–8 ounces of purified warm water and drink first thing in the morning. Wait 15–30 minutes before eating or drinking anything else. This is great for a quick liver flush and to get the juices flowing.

- Instead of buying flavored water, most of which are loaded with sugar, make your own flavored water either by adding lemon or lime or by adding 2 cups of fruit to 1 gallon of water and drinking it throughout the day. Use by the end of the next day.

- Add a 1/4 teaspoon of ground turmeric to a few ounces of purified warm water and drink. This is almost a cure-all but is especially helpful in reducing inflammation. For cold climates, add a pinch of ground ginger with the turmeric in the winter.

- Use coriander (ground, seeds, or leaves [cilantro]) for a cooling effect. This is especially helpful to use with nightshades and spicy food if they give you trouble.

- If you tolerate dairy, drink 1 cup of warm milk with 1 teaspoon of ghee to help relax before bedtime. Be sure to rotate, having it no more than once every four days.

- For a healthier margarita, squeeze 1/2–1 lime into a shot of high-quality tequila. Add stevia if you need some sweetness. Mix well and sip. The higher quality alcohol used, the less sweetener and other stuff you need to add to make it taste good. I'm not advocating alcohol, but if you do have a mixed drink occasionally, there are ways to make it easier on your body. In the case of mixed drinks, it's often the sugar and drink mixes that are more offensive to the body than the alcohol. Notice how both the alcohol and the sugar affect you.

- Store fresh herbs such as parsley and cilantro in a vase or glass of water in the refrigerator covered loosely with a plastic bag. They'll stay fresh longer, up to 2 weeks, so you won't keep running out.

- As a substitute for egg, try mixing 1 tablespoon of chia seeds with 3 tablespoons of water, let it sit for ten minutes, and then add to a recipe as you would 1 egg. Double the amount to substitute for 2 eggs. It may not work as well for a recipe with more than 2 eggs. Flax seeds can also be used.

- Another substitute for egg is a ripe banana. About 1/4–1/2 a ripe banana can be substituted for 1 egg in muffin recipes and some other baked goods. Again, this works well when the recipe calls for 1 or 2 eggs and may not work as well if more than 2 eggs are called for.

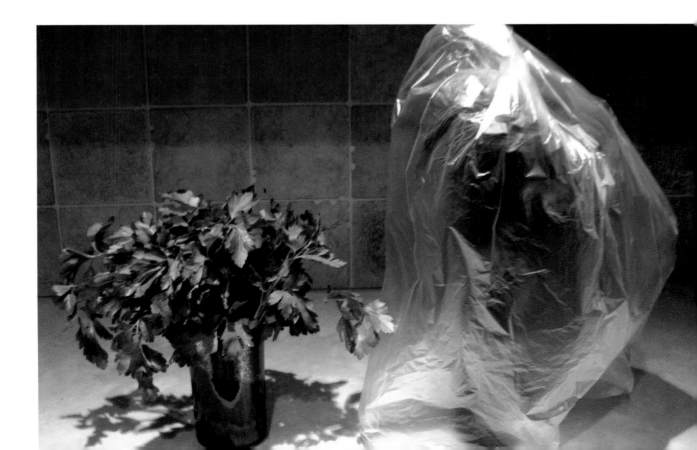

SIX FOUNDATION PRINCIPLES TO LIVE A HEALTHY LIFE

Diet

If diet is wrong, medicine is of no use. If diet is correct, medicine is of no need.
—Ayurvedic proverb

To live in balance and good health, one must address all aspects of oneself. What we put in our bodies is a great place to start. Food is very personal, more so than I ever realized. There is absolute truth to the saying, "One man's medicine is another man's poison." I've seen and experienced many people use food to control others. I witness, almost daily, people relegating their food choices to others. I've learned the hard way (it feels good to say this out loud), "Only I should decide what goes into my body, no matter how reputable the restaurant, experienced the chef, or dear the relative." Be your own detective and decision-maker. Get creative, take your time, and take control. There are unlimited ways to accommodate your needs without causing a commotion or inconveniencing anyone. Eat what nourishes you, and enjoy.

Hydration

Adequate hydration is crucial to overall health. Chronic dehydration (getting less than adequate amounts of water on a regular basis) can elicit feelings of hunger, causing people to eat when they should drink and causing or perpetuating ailments and diseases such as dry skin, hypertension, migraines, allergies, and arthritis. Experts recommend drinking half your body weight (pounds) in ounces per day. For example, if you weigh 150 pounds you should drink 75 ounces of purified water per day; not herbal tea, carbonated flavored water, or coconut water, but pure water (1 liter = 33.8 ounces). This amount is for a typical day, and more water may be needed if you have a hard, sweaty workout that day. I prefer to drink flat mineral water so I don't dilute too many minerals from my body, but any water free of chemicals such as chlorine is a good place to start (avoid tap water unless it's filtered). Also, avoid distilled water, as it is completely devoid of minerals and will quickly demineralize you, which can also cause dehydration. As I first learned in my college endocrinology class, the balance of water and salts in our body is an important and delicate one. Maintain this balance by drinking mineral water (or you can add a pinch of sea salt to your purified tap or spring water to add some minerals back in).

Sleep

Do you want to know the secret to longevity? Sleep. Adequate sleep can also help you lose weight by balancing hormones. Each person may vary slightly, but it is generally recommended to sleep between the hours of 10:00 p.m. and 6:00 a.m. These hours allow us to harmonize with the rhythm of nature by sleeping when it gets dark and waking with the sun. There have been numerous studies showing the importance of getting enough sleep before midnight, which many of us do not do. Sleep is when we regenerate, rejuvenate, and repair our body and mind. Lack of sleep leads to nonoptimal function to varying degrees. Some experts say that our physical body repairs during the hours of 10:00 p.m. and 2:00 a.m. and our mind and emotional state repairs and rejuvenates during the hours of 2:00 a.m. and 6:00 a.m. Which one are you shortchanging? Does it show? It does for me when I get to bed too late, which is still something I do far too often.

Breathing

If you've ever watched a baby breathe, you probably noticed that the baby's abdomen moved, not the chest. A newborn baby innately knows how to breathe naturally; the breath beginning from the diaphragm and not the chest. Once a fear or trauma occurs in a person's life, he/she may respond by holding his/her breath. When these patterns of fear or stress happen again and again, we begin to form a habit of shallow chest breathing. To relearn the natural relaxing and revitalizing diaphragmatic breath, we can practice yoga, meditation, Qi Gong, or simply try deep breathing by placing one hand on your abdomen and one on your chest to see which one moves when you inhale. Ideally, your abdomen should expand when you inhale and retract when you exhale. Your chest will rise on the inhale, too, but this should happen after your abdomen expands. A deep diaphragmatic breath sends your body the message that everything is okay and you can relax. Shallow breathing, like that which would occur during a stressful situation, sends the fight or flight message and releases stress hormones. Constant shallow breathing plays a role in keeping you in a chronic stress response. Proper, rhythmic, diaphragmatic breathing helps to maintain homeostasis and a relaxed state. Try taking three or more deep, diaphragmatic breaths right now and notice how you feel.

Thoughts

One of my favorite local eateries has a plaque on the counter that says, "Change your thoughts, and you change your world." I've experienced this to be true and amazing. We can eat the healthiest food, drink adequate water, and get plenty of rest, but if we are filled with negative, self-defeating thoughts we will not reach our optimal health, and we may even send ourselves into a disease state. I invite you to become aware of that voice in your subconscious that scolds you for being wrong or tells you you're not good enough to achieve your dream. The voice that constantly reminds you of that "to do" list that remains undone, makes up stories concerning other people, or thinks everyone else is an inconsiderate idiot, especially if they're driving anywhere near you. When you notice this voice, smile and acknowledge it. Then dismiss it and think of another way to look at that same scenario. We all have a defeatist voice at times, which is normal, but you must find balance. Ask yourself, "What do I believe?" Do I believe that the world is generally a good place full of good people, or do I believe people suck, life sucks, and then you die? Your outlook and beliefs have a powerful effect on your organs, your stress response, and your overall health and well-being. Change your thoughts, and you change your world.

Movement

Moving your body every day will keep things flowing. And, "If it ain't movin' it's dyin,'" as my chiropractor says. I am not suggesting that you force yourself to spend 30 minutes on a treadmill every day, especially if you dread it. Find something you like and do that. It can be running, weightlifting, paddling, boxing, or it can be dancing or walking around the city. And here's the fun part, for every workout you do, you get to do a work-in. A workout is when you expend energy, exerting yourself to the point of an elevated heart rate and sweating. A work-in is when you take in energy and feel relaxed and rejuvenated afterward. What if we kept withdrawing money from our bank account without depositing money? We'd soon be depleted. What if we keep expending energy but not replenishing energy? We'll end up depleted. So when you're feeling exhausted and low on energy, the last thing you should do is expend what little energy you have at the gym. Instead try some Qi Gong, T'ai Chi, yoga, or a relaxing walk. And when you're feeling jittery or like you need to blow off steam, it's a great time for a workout. If you can't decide which to do or you're attached to your workout schedule, at least try adding in a few minutes of working-in each time you work out. It can be immediately after your workout or later that day. Either way, it will replenish your body's energy stores.

Note: I'd like to credit Paul Chek as the original thinker who organized the concept of *The Six Foundation Principles* under yin/yang headings (always in dynamic balance). Please go to http://chekinstitute.com/ to learn more.

All of these topics and more can be further explored at Energize Body & Mind, LLC. For more information, please visit www.EnergizeBodyandMind.com.

RESOURCES

Recommended Food Brands

trüRoots (sprouted legumes)

Navitas Naturals (navitasnaturals.com)

Manitoba Harvest Hemp Foods (ManitobaHarvest.com)

Explore Asian (mung bean and black bean pasta)

King Soba (buckwheat noodles)

Gold Mine (kelp noodles)

Sea Seasonings (dulse)

Columbia River Organics (when frozen vegetables are needed)

Bionaturae fruit spread (Bionaturae.com)

Bob's Red Mill (organic and gluten-free flours)

Muraca chestnut flour

Love'n Bake almond paste

Minerve chestnut purée

Clement Faugier chestnut purée

Pacific mushroom broth (For chicken, beef, and vegetable broth, choose the brand with purest ingredients. I've found that it's not always Pacific brand in these cases.)

Paleo wraps (Pure coconut wraps. I've found them in a few health food stores as well as on-line at Amazon and ThriveMarke.)

I buy most of these products at my local health food grocery store. Whole Foods also has many of these foods, and Amazon.com often has difficult-to-find food brands and products.

Online Food Shopping Resources

Nuts.com

iHerb.com

Honeyville.com

Longevitywarehouse.com

Julianbakery.com

Paleowrap.com

Amazon.com

Thrivemarket.com

Helpful and Informative Food Websites

Theorganicfoodguide.com

Localharvest.org

Greenpeople.org

Eatwild.com

Grassfedbeefrestaurants.com

Grassfedtraditions.com

Gmo-awareness.com

Calorieking.com/foods

RESOURCES

Ayurvedic Cooking for Self-Healing by Usha and Dr. Vasant Lad, 1997. The Ayurvedic Institute, P.O. Box 23445, Albuquerque, NM 87192-1445, (505) 291-9698

Eat-Taste-Heal by Thomas Yarema, MD, Daniel Rhoda, Johnny Brannigan

How to Eat, Move, and be Healthy! by Paul Chek

Know Your Fats: The Complete Primer for Understanding the Nutrition of Fats, Oils, and Cholesterol by Mary G. Enig, Ph.D, 2000

Ayurveda.com

chekinstitute.com

RECOMMENDED READING

How to Eat, Move, and be Healthy! by Paul Chek

Wheat Belly by Dr. William Davis

Clean by Alejandro Junger, MD

Yang, Q. "Gain Weight by 'going diet?'" Artificial Sweeteners and the Neurobiology of Sugar Cravings. *Yale J Biol Med.* Jun 2010; 83(2): 101–108

Your Body's Many Cries for Water by F. Batmanghelidj, MD

INDEX

80/20 rule 22

A

ADD/ADHD 25

Addiction 21,23

Alcohol 16, 21, 188

All-Day carrot pancakes 174

Allergy 11, 25

Almond cake 180

Almond milk 162, 172, 175

Almond pancakes 172

Almond smoothie 167

Alzheimer's 25

Apple crisp 181

Anxiety 16

Arctic char with capers and dill 55

Aromatic granola 158, 159

Artichokes, stuffed 13, 83

Artificial sweeteners 16, 22, 24, 196

Asparagus, simply cooked 82, 93

Autism 25

Ayurveda 14, 17, 90, 196

B

Baby back ribs 75

Balanced eggplant 89

Beef

    Beef stew 76

    Grass-fed filet mignon 68

    Grass-fed steak tips 69, 76

    Pot roast 78

    Twisted tacos 71

Beets in balsamic dressing 96

Bloating 16, 18

Brain fog 16

Breakfast

    All-day carrot pancakes 174

    Almond pancakes 172

    Breakfast popover 175

    Cashew smoothie 166

    Coconut almond smoothie 167

    Coconut berry smoothie 165

    Infamous green smoothie 169

    Mehul's nutty pancakes 171

    Pumpkin pancakes 173

    Savory omelet 170

    Scones 176

Breakfast popover 175

Brussels sprouts 92

Buckwheat noodles in ginger garlic sauce 130

Butter 17, 31, 37, 41

Butternut squash soup 138

C

Caffeine 16

Calamari, sautéed 61

Carrot ginger soup 136

Carrot pancakes 174

Casein 17

Cashew milk 163

Cashew smoothie 166

Celery root chips 99

Celiac disease 25, 27

Chestnut cookies178

Chicken, lemon 66

Chicken, roasted with root vegetables 79

Chicken wings, dry rub 64, 65

Chimichurri sauce 47, 144

Chocolate, warm cakes 183

Chocolate delights, dark 178, 180, 186

Cholesterol 29, 30, 196

Clogged sinuses 16

Coconut 17, 21, 31, 37, 38, 39, 104, 185

Coconut almond smoothie 167

Coconut berry smoothie 165

Coconut carob candies 185

Cod with Moroccan spices 53

Colorful spring salad 102

Constipation 16

Corn 16, 21, 28, 31, 40, 41

Cramps 16, 19

Cranberry sauce 147

Cravings 22, 23, 196

Creamy greens dressing 151

Crohn's disease 25

D

Dairy-free 11, 17, 42

Dark Chocolate Delights 186

Depression 25

Desserts

    Almond cake 180

    Apple crisp 181

    Chestnut cookies 178

    Coconut carob candies 185

    Dark Chocolate Delights 186

    Tapioca 182

    Warm Chocolate cakes 183

Detox 15, 29

Dhana Jiru 36, 46, 88

Diet 5, 11, 14-17, 21, 22, 25-31, 33, 42, 90, 190, 196

Digestion 18

Dijon Kale and Squash 112

Dressings

    Creamy Greens 151

    Mango-Lime 150

    Old-Fashioned, in Fashion,
        Lemon and Olive Oil 150

    Orange-Ginger 151

Dry cough 16

E

Eggplant, balanced 89

Egg substitute 189

Eggs 16

Elimination Diet 11, 16, 17, 26, 42

Emotional eating 23

Endive with Blue Cheese 155

Energy 5, 12, 29, 30, 41, 192, 193

Essentials for the pantry 35

F

Fats 17, 29-32

Fertility 29

Filet mignon, grass-fed 68

Fish

    Arctic char with capers and dill 55

    Cod with Moroccan spices 53

    Haddock and vegetables in foil 48

    Haddock with fresh salsa 50

    Hake with Chimichurri 47

    Fish filets with olive tapenade and lemon 51

    New moon salmon 56

    Red fish with roasted radicchio and spinach 58

    Sardines 38, 153, 154

    Sautéed calamari 61

    Tuna steaks 46

    Tuna tartare 62

Food combining 18

Food elimination 11, 16, 17, 26, 42

Food intolerance 15, 16, 26

Food rotation 15, 90
Foundation principles 190-193
Fresh Calamari 61
Fresh potato salad with green beans 119
Fresh tomato sauce 145
Frittata 108
Fun food and kitchen tips 188
Fungal Infection 23

G

Gas 16, 18
Ghee 17, 31, 37
Gluten 11, 16, 17, 22, 25-28, 30, 38, 42
Gluten-free (GF) 11, 17, 25-28, 38, 42
Grains 16, 25, 27, 28, 31, 42
Granola 153, 158
Grass-fed filet mignon 68
Grass-fed steak tips 69, 76
Graves' disease 25
Green beans in fresh potato salad 119
Green beans with mustard dressing 94
Greens, sautéed 91
Greens wrapped in coconut 104
Guacamole 153, 156

H

Haddock and fresh salsa 50
Haddock and vegetables in foil 48
Hake with chimichurri 47
Hashimoto's 25
Healthy lifestyle 190
Heavy hitters 16
Hemp milk 164
Herbed turkey thighs 74
Herb storage 189
Hormones 29, 30, 191, 192
Hyperactivity 20

I

Infamous green smoothie 169
Inflammation 20, 25, 29, 188
Intolerance 15-17, 25, 26
Irritability 16

J

Joint aches and pains 16, 26

K

Kale, Dijon squash 112
Kelp noodle, raw salad 132
Kelp noodle stir-fry 111
Khichadi, mung dal 126

L

Lack of focus 16
Lactose 17, 24
Lamb lollipops 67
Lemon chicken 66
Lentils, khichadi, macro trio, red, soup 108, 126, 128, 139
Lethargy 16
Lifestyle tips 190
Liver flush 188
Lucky Lentil Soup 139

M

Mango-Lime dressing 150
Margarita, healthier version 188
Meat
    Baby back ribs 75
    Beef stew 76
    Chicken wings with dry rub 64, 65
    Grass-fed filet mignon 68
    Grass-fed steak tips 69

Herbed turkey thighs 74
Lamb lollipops 67
Lemon chicken 66
Pot roast 78
Roasted chicken and root vegetables 79
Sesame pork chops 72
Twisted tacos 71
Mehul's nutty pancakes 171
Metabolic type 17, 21
Multiple sclerosis 25
Mung dal khichadi 126
Mushroom soup 134
Mushrooms 17, 100

N

New moon salmon 56
Nightshades 17, 114, 188
Nut-free 11, 17, 42
Nuts 11, 16, 17, 31, 37, 41

O

Ode to my Italian heritage: Stuffed artichokes 83
Oils 17, 31, 32, 40, 41
Old-fashioned, in fashion, lemon, and olive oil 150
Okra 87
Orange-ginger dressing 151
Organic 10, 11, 21, 22, 31, 37, 38, 40, 41

P

Pain 16, 26
Pancakes
    All-day carrot 147
    Almond 172
    Mehul's nutty 171
    Pumpkin 173
Peanuts 16
Peppers, sautéed 98

Peppers, stuffed 85
Pesto Risotto 124
Pesto sauce 143
Popover, breakfast 175
Pork (sesame chops, baby back ribs) 72, 75
Portabella mushrooms 100
Potato salad, fresh with green beans 119
Potato, roasted with sage 121
Pot roast 78
Poultry (dry rub chicken wings, lemon chicken, herbed
    turkey thighs, roasted chicken) 64, 66, 74, 79
Pumpkin pancakes 173
Puttanesca Sauce 146

Q

Quick tips 33
Quinoa, spiced 122
Quinoa, with greens 116

R

Radicchio, red fish and spinach 58
Radicchio with fennel 95
Raw kelp noodle salad 132
Red fish with roasted radicchio and spinach 58
Red lentils 128
Ribs, slow cooked baby back 75
Risotto, pesto 124
Rheumatoid arthritis 25
Roasted chicken with root vegetables 79

S

Salad Dressings
    Creamy greens dressing 151
    Old-fashioned, in fashion, lemon, and olive oil
        150
    Orange-ginger dressing 151
    Mango-lime dressing 150

Salads
    Colorful spring salad 102
    Fresh potato salad with green beans 119
    Sicilian Fennel and Orange salad 103
    Spiced Quinoa salad 122
    Suzanne's peppery floral salad 101
Saffron rice 117
Sage potatoes 121
Salmon, new moon 56
Salsa Verde 157
Salt 19, 20, 36, 42
Sardines 38, 153, 154
Sauces
    Chimichurri 144
    Cranberry sauce 147
    Fresh tomato sauce 145
    Pesto 143
    Puttanesca 146
Sautéed calamari 61
Sautéed greens 91
Sautéed peppers 98
Savory omelet 170
Schizophrenia 25
Scones 176
Seeds 16, 31, 37, 188, 189
Sesame pork chops 72
Shellfish 16
Sicilian fennel and orange salad 103
Sinuses 16
Six foundation principles 190
Skin rashes 16
Slow cooked baby back ribs 75
Smoothies
    Cashew smoothie 166
    Coconut almond smoothie 167
    Coconut berry smoothie 165
    Infamous green smoothie 169
Snacks
    Aromatic granola 153, 158

Endive with Blue Cheese 155
    Guacamole 153, 156
    Salsa Verde 157
    Sardines 153, 154
Spiced quinoa salad 122
Spiced vegetable stew 114
Spices 22, 36, 40
Soups
    Butternut squash soup 138
    Carrot ginger soup 136
    Lucky lentil soup 139
    Mushroom soup 134
Soy 16, 40, 41
Soy-free 11, 17, 42
Spiced Quinoa 122
Spiced vegetable stew 114
Steak tips, grass fed 69
Steak, tuna 46
Stevia 21, 39, 153, 188
Stew
    Beef stew 76
    Spiced vegetable stew 114
Squash, Dijon kale and 112
Stuffed artichokes 13, 83
Stuffed peppers 85
Sugar 16, 17, 20-24, 27, 29, 152, 153, 188, 196
Suzanne's peppery floral salad 101

T

Tapioca 182
Tips 33, 188, 190
Toxins/toxicity 29, 30
Traditional and so simple pot roast 78
Tuna Steaks 46
Tuna tartare over arugula 62
Turkey, herbed thighs 74
Twisted taco 71

V

Vegetables
    Asparagus, simply cooked 82, 93
    Balanced eggplant 89
    Beets in balsamic dressing 96
    Brussels sprouts 92
    Celery root chips 99
    Dijon kale and squash 112
    Green beans with mustard dressing 94
    Greens wrapped in coconut 104
    Okra 87
    Radicchio with fennel 95
    Sautéed greens 91
    Sautéed peppers 98
    Stuffed artichoke 13, 83
    Zucchini, Indian style 88

Vegetarian
    Buckwheat noodles in ginger garlic sauce 130
    Squash soup 138
    Carrot ginger soup 136
    Fresh potato salad with green beans 119
    Frittata 108
    Greens wrapped in coconut 104
    Kelp noodle stir-fry 111
    Mung dal khichadi 126
    Mushroon soup 134
    Pesto risotto 124
    Portabella mushrooms 100
    Quinoa with greens 116
    Raw kelp noodle salad 132
    Red lentils 128
    Saffron rice 117
    Sage potatoes 121
    Spiced quinoa salad 122
    Spiced vegetable stew 114
    Vegetarian macro trio 109

W

Warm chocolate cakes 183
Water 41, 190, 191
Weekend recipes
    Beef stew 76
    Herbed turkey thighs 74
    Pot roast 78
    Roasted chicken with root vegetables 79
    Slow-cooked baby back ribs 75
Weight loss (as side effect) 25, 26
Wheat 13, 16, 25-28
Whey 17

X

Xylitol 21

Y

Yeast 16, 20

Z

Zucchini, Indian style 88

PERSONAL OPTIMAL HEALTH NOTES

PERSONAL OPTIMAL
HEALTH NOTES

PERSONAL OPTIMAL HEALTH NOTES

PERSONAL OPTIMAL
HEALTH NOTES

PERSONAL OPTIMAL HEALTH NOTES

PERSONAL OPTIMAL HEALTH NOTES